Sharon Moore has done a great service for people with lupus, and for all people suffering with a chronic disease. She has written a very useful and informative book that can serve as a roadmap back to health. It should be read by those who are ill and by the practitioners they choose to work with. . . . The information and explanations presented are the pearls from thousands of dollars worth of consultations with many different types of practitioners.

John Ruhland, N.D., Bastyr University

Lupus: Alternative Therapies That Work is a book I recommend to not only those with lupus, but to anyone with a disease that is difficult to categorize or treat. It is the story of the author's journey through a painful and confusing disease process, and it is a success story because of her own strength and persistence. . . . This is a book about life and all its possibilities, and the rewards that come from a commitment to healing. **Eric Steese, Ph.D., Clinical Psychologist**

Sharon Moore has eloquently documented her journey with lupus. She describes the therapies that helped in her recovery and gives rationales for each treatment. Particularly helpful is a twelve-month plan for incorporating these varied therapies into a lifestyle that optimally supports recovery and personal growth.

Pamela Houghton, N.D., L.Ac.

From the terrifying opening to the "clues" that lead to her own recovery [Sharon Moore's *Lupus*] reads like the best kind of detective story—one where the case is solved through tenacity, intelligence, and compassion. There's a wealth of good information about alternative medicine in this book and Sharon's message of hope shines through every page.

Rosemary Jones, HealingPgs.com, online bookstore for alternative medicine

Ms. Moore gives the reader both scientific and historical background with an upbeat, informative, compassionate, and spiritual flair. . . . *Lupus: Alternative Therapies That Work* may well be the most valuable reference material for providing the information needed to care for oneself. . . . Ms. Moore has shown that taking her power back has helped her to feel better and given her hope for life beyond lupus—it could well do the same for others.

George J. Grobins, D.D.S., P.S.

Lupus

ALTERNATIVE

THERAPIES

THAT WORK

Sharon Moore

Healing Arts Press
Rochester, Vermont

Healing Arts Press
One Park Street
Rochester, Vermont 05767
www.InnerTraditions.com

Healing Arts Press is a division of Inner Traditions International

*Note to the reader: This book is intended as an informational guide. The remedies,
approaches, and techniques described herein are meant to supplement, and not to be a
substitute for, professional medical care or treatment. They should not be used to treat a
serious ailment without prior consultation with a qualified health care professional.*

Library of Congress Cataloging-in-Publication Data
Moore, Sharon.
    Lupus : alternative therapies that work / Sharon Moore.
        p. cm.
    Includes bibliographical references and index.
    ISBN 0-89281-889-1 (alk. paper)
    1. Systemic lupus erythematosus—Alternative treatment. I. Title.

    RC924.5.L85 M66 2000
    616.7'7—dc21

                                                        00-040843

Printed and bound in the United States

10 9 8 7 6 5 4 3 2 1

Text design and layout by Wendy Pratt
This book was typeset in Minion

*Although the author quotes numerous animal studies in the context
of this book, she would like her readers to know that she considers the
use of animals in medical experiments to be inhumane.*

Contents

To my husband, Steve, and my parents,
Muriel and Don,
who never stopped believing
that I would recover from lupus.

Acknowledgments

Many people participated directly and indirectly in the creation of this book. To each of them I extend my deep gratitude for their assistance and compasssion over the long years of my recovery and the writing of this manuscript.

Marion Waby encouraged me to write about my healing process. Ruth Ann Londardelli spent many hours reading and discussing the manuscript with me. Librarians Patty Bergman, Rosalie Spellman, Pat Matheny-White, and Jay Windisck provided research assistance. My agent, Joshua Bilmes, found an excellent home for the book with Healing Arts Press. Book project editor Elaine Sanborn was a skilled and patient teacher.

Friends and family played a vital role in helping me stay connected with the world when I was suffering with a debilitating illness. They are: Jonnie Kae Anderson, Reverend Don Bernard, Harry Bowron, Sharri Faulkner Boyd, Kathleen Cannon, Barbara Cashion, Jo Curtz, Terry Curry, Joel Davis, D. J. Delaney, Carol DeMent, Karen and Bob Dick, Rollie Geppart, Barbara Gilles, Velma Grigsby, Jane Hall, Trisha Hamilton, Tim Haralson, Rosana and Kelly Hart, Betty Hauser, Rich Henry, Danny and Anna Hernandez, June Kersog-Hinson, Joe, Yolanda, Janiva, Sonja, and Chago Cifuentes-Hiss, Jackie Huetter, Rosemary Jones, Lorna Joslin, John and Dorothy Killian, Deb Langhans, Doris and Clayt Larsen, Reverend Sandra Lee, Don and Peggy Levine, Marilyn Lewis, Pia and David Lozier, Blanche Mailhot, Susan Meline, Lucia Miltenberger, Dr. Michael Moore, the Peeples family, Sue, Julie, and Nicole Peters, Ruth Pevey, Rick and Cindy Quam, Laura Ralph, Kim Riano, Bob and Alletia Simons, Don and Carol Stubb, Geshe Jamyang Sultrim, Susan Tepper, Patty Thoe and Terry Hogan,

Samantha and Rachel Schechter-Thoe, Carol Trasatto, Susan Wallace, Bermaht and Phil Wampler, Jan Wiesenfeld, Barbara Williamson, Kathleen and Chris Wolfe, and Joan Zappetini.

A team of compassionate health care professionals guided me on my journey back to health. They included: Suzanne Adams, N.D., Liliane Bartha, M.D., David Buscher, M.D., Qiang Cao, L.Ac., Sherwin Cottler, Ph.D., Walter Crinnion, N.D., Sandra Denton, M.D., Pamela Houghton, N.D., Steve Kirkpatrick, D.D.S., Mary McCanna, M.A., Robin Moore, N.D., Eric Steese, Ph.D., Jonathan Wright, M.D., and Bing Zhou, L.Ac.

Introduction

This is the story of my recovery from systemic lupus erythematosus (SLE) using alternative therapies. It is the story of my healing from an illness so deep, so encompassing, that my survival seemed unlikely. It is the story of my discovery of my own healing resources. It is also the story of the compassionate alternative health practitioners who helped me.

Fourteen years ago, in the middle of my "mystery" illness, I made the choice of treating my debilitating symptoms with alternative medicine. I hoped to avoid the potentially serious, long-term effects of the pharmaceuticals my doctors wanted to use to treat my symptoms, so I began a search through health care practices that hover outside the boundaries of conventional Western medicine. Five years into that long and difficult process, I was finally diagnosed with systemic lupus erythematosus. By then, I had found alternative therapies from other cultures and other perspectives within my own culture that were helping me. Over time, those therapies have healed most of the lupus symptoms that plagued me for so long.

This book offers an account of what I've learned about self-care and alternative treatments for lupus. Various applications of naturopathy, nutritional medicine, traditional Chinese medicine, nontoxic dentistry, environmental medicine, and energy medicine have helped me. The information and suggestions I present here do not guarantee recovery. Nevertheless, if you have a mild to moderate case of systemic lupus erythematosus, I hope this book will empower you to begin managing your illness using some of the alternative therapies I discuss. As a lupus patient, you have a right to know about treatments spanning the whole healing spectrum that may help you regain your health.

1

My Story

There is only one journey. Going inside yourself.

Rainer Maria Rilke

"What's wrong with me?" My eyes sweep the inner city hospital emergency room as I lie very still. What began as a pleasant holiday for my husband, Steve, and me, at the 1986 World's Fair in Vancouver, Canada, has plummeted into terror. It's 10 p.m. The bright overhead lights of the room burn my eyes. Ambulance sirens signal injury and suffering. The screams and sobs of ill and wounded people ricochet through the rooms. The man next to me moans with acute food poisoning. Two beds away a gunshot victim whimpers as a police officer guards him.

This is not my idea of a holiday. I've been lying here for hours now, terrified and exhausted. After endless waiting, I'm still hoping the doctors can give me a diagnosis for this mystery illness. Over and over I review the day, my mind stuck on details, searching for clues to what has happened to me. After viewing the international exhibits at the Vancouver's 1986 World Exposition, Steve and I dined on chicken and kimchi in a Korean restaurant on the exposition grounds. Following dinner, we entered the U.S. pavilion. Standing on a conveyor that carried us through a large darkened room, we were watching a colorful collage of American life on several slide screens.

Then, quite suddenly, I felt as though the room were closing in on me. My heart began pounding wildly. The room began to swirl. I groped through the crowd gasping, "Excuse me, excuse me, I've got to get out." People pressed aside as I staggered toward the neon exit sign. Lunging through the door, I collapsed on the pavement outside. Steve found me moments later dripping with perspiration, struggling for breath and babbling, "Get me some help. Please help me."

Still lying on the gurney in the emergency room, I see the doctors approaching. I can feel my apprehension as one doctor leans over me, touching my shoulder gently. "After all the tests we've run," she says, "we can't find anything wrong with you. We think you may have just an acute case of panic. Nothing to worry about. This sometimes happens to people in large crowds. You'll be fine tomorrow." "Panic?" I say, not comprehending. "Is that what this is? Panic?" I've never experienced anything so awful in my life. I can barely breathe. I'm so weak and dizzy that I can't stand up. I'm afraid to let go of my husband or the nurses. I feel as if the bottom is falling out of my brain, out of my stomach, out of my life. "If this is panic," I say, "what on earth is causing it?"

Discharged from the hospital the next morning, I sat next to Steve as we drove back to our home in Olympia, Washington. We talked about the strange, unnerving episode and agreed that it was best to put it behind us. I expected to recover quickly and go on with my life. But that was not to be. We could never have imagined that this emergency room episode in Vancouver was the harbinger of five years of deepening illness, followed by seven more years of agonizingly slow recovery. There would be countless "panic attacks," more emergency room visits, a long hospitalization, and years of illness that continued to mystify the doctors.

Shortly after the Vancouver incident, I began to realize that I was having difficulty driving. The road seemed to be coming up at me. Working as a vocational rehabilitation counselor, I was seeing severely disabled clients over a three-county area, and I needed to drive a lot. One sunny afternoon I was heading north on the freeway to Seattle to set up a college training program for a client. As I was passing a military base, I suddenly felt as if all the traffic were coming straight at me. I broke into a cold sweat, my mouth went dry, and I began to lose my peripheral vision. It seemed as if I might be close to blacking out.

Swerving onto the nearest exit ramp, I curved around to a military checkpoint, where I stopped and told one of the guards, "I'm very ill. Can you make a phone call for me?" "No, ma'am," he answered. "We can't help you. Drive on. There are cars behind you waiting to get into the base." What to do? I thought I had only a short time left before I blacked out. I was beginning to hyperventilate and was trying to concentrate on breathing more slowly to give myself a few more seconds of consciousness.

In the forest ahead I glimpsed a large pink building. Driving into the parking lot, I got shakily out of the car and staggered inside. Suddenly surrounded by mirrors, glistening bodies, and rock music, I realized that I must be in an athletic club. "Please," I blurted out to a man wearing a badge that read "Trainer." "I'm ill and I'm blacking out. . . ." That is all I can recall. When I awoke, I was lying on a blanket outside, a pillow under my head, and my golden retriever, T.G., who had been riding with me, nuzzling my face. Medics in blue uniforms leaned over me.

"Ma'am, how are you now? Can you sit up?"

"No," I said. " The trees are swirling terribly, and I'm very weak. Can you please call my husband to come and get me?"

"Ma'am, we're going to need to take you in the ambulance to the hospital. Your blood pressure is very high, and your eyes are dilated. Are you a drug addict?"

The question shocked me. "I'm not on drugs," I insisted. "But I'm very ill. I've got to find out what's wrong with me."

So another ambulance delivered me to another hospital emergency room. "Just breathe into this paper bag for a while, and you'll be fine," the intern was saying. At this point I became angry. "Look, I could have passed out on the freeway and been killed or killed someone else. I could have died at that athletic club. And you're telling me to breathe into a paper bag and I'll be fine? I can't seem to get any help in these hospitals. I want to know what this illness is."

The technician explained that my system was overly oxygenated from my rapid breathing. By breathing into the paper bag, I was inhaling my own carbon dioxide, which would rebalance my blood oxygen levels. But what was causing my "panic?" I asked. It seemed to come from nowhere. The technician answered that they had no idea about what causes panic. He drew blood and ordered laboratory tests, all of which showed negative results. Once again I left a hospital emergency room with no answers, hoping that whatever was terrorizing me would go away and let me live a normal life again.

Over subsequent months I was visited with more so-called panic attacks, and I began to feel physically ill. I had reached a point where I could no longer drive. I also had lost the intellectual ability to write the complex rehabilitation plans my work required. Forced to quit my job, I was so ill that I could barely get to doctors' appointments. When I could barely manage to get out of bed, we searched for a doctor to make a house call. No one would come. Finally, a young American medical doctor who had trained in France agreed to visit. After a cursory examination, he announced that I didn't have a life-threatening disease, but he didn't know what it was. We wondered how he knew it wasn't life-threatening when he couldn't diagnose it. My family was so worried about my deteriorating condition that they begged him to hospitalize me. Resisting at first, he finally listened to our pleas and arranged to admit me to a hospital.

By this time I was so weak that I could not feed myself. My vision was impaired to the point that I could not read. I could barely hear people talking to me. I could not think clearly. When I talked, I knew I wasn't making sense. I burned with a persistent fever. Constant pain shot through my muscles and joints. My body moaned with deep fatigue. Nights brought the dread of insomnia, hallucinations, nightmares, dry mouth and eyes. I had severe periodontal disease and lost thirty-five pounds. I also experienced nausea; heart palpitations; eczema on my stomach, knees, and hands; and a large, fluted rash on my face. During that hospitalization, my family knew that I was so ill I might die. They hugged me, cried, and prayed. How had this happened to their once strong, vibrant daughter? What was this terrible illness? Steve moved into the hospital room with me, holding me through long hours of my semi-consciousness.

There, in a stark, fourth-floor hospital room high above the Douglas fir forests I love, I lay watching seagulls and an occasional blue heron soar against the pearly swirl of clouds. I imagined myself soaring with them and, for a time, forgot the illness that wracked my body and mind. The three attending doctors rarely came to see me and carried out few tests. But the nurses handed me many drugs and insisted on watching me swallow them. They didn't tell me what those pharmaceuticals were, all of which made me more sick. My family saw me growing worse and became even more alarmed. One of my nurses had worked in Mexican and French hospitals. She told me that medical care, in her opinion, was much better in those countries than in the United States. I could tell she was concerned about all the medications she was required to give me. Finally, one morning I told her I could not take any more drugs. She nodded in agreement, her mouth set, and watched as I flushed the pills down the toilet.

During this time, the strange rash on my left cheek alarmed my father. Both of us pointed it out to the doctors. One doctor said that it was indeed unusual and then continued to ignore it. Every day the doctors wanted to send me home. Every day I resisted. "Please let me stay," I begged. "I'm so ill that I'm afraid to go home. My family is concerned that they can't take care of me." After nine days in my arboreal room above the soft, reflective grayness of Puget Sound, I was required to leave. We still had no diagnosis. Steve pushed me in a wheelchair toward our car and drove me home. There I languished, my weakness growing more foreboding and the rash that looked like a butterfly still a frozen flutter on my left cheek.

As I lay in bed at home, by now utterly debilitated, I wondered over and over how this had happened to me. How had I become so weak, so sick, so terrified? Was there a cause of this illness somewhere in my background? I recalled going out to East Africa in the 1960s as a Peace Corps volunteer to work as an English teacher in Uganda. I was excited to arrive at the school compound in northwestern Uganda where I was to work for two years. Built by the Christian Missionary Society in the early 1900s, the school served for decades as a boarding school exclusively for Christian students. Uganda's independence in 1962 allowed the new government to confiscate private schools. They intended to provide universal education for the first time to all Ugandan youth. The country needed volunteer teachers to fill in until they could train enough teachers to staff all their schools. I felt privileged to offer my teaching skills to a society that was trying to learn what it is to be free.

Our old school buildings were molded of mud and full of white ants— a kind of termite—munching the structures slowly to the ground. I lived two hundred yards away in an ancient, ten-room, colonial-style, mud-and-brick house. A lovely place, it had large rooms, wide-screened windows, and a covered veranda. One evening shortly after I arrived, as I was correcting papers by lantern light at my desk near a window, a dark shadow padded across the veranda. My God, I thought, that was a lion. Yes, it was a lion, and I was truly in Africa.

At night, small lizards called geckos sometimes lost their grip on the ceiling above my bed and plopped on my face, awakening me. As I tried to glide back into sleep, I could hear the white ants cracking mud in their jaws in the wall near my pillowed head. They were working methodically at eating my house to the ground, too.

We were living in a malaria region, and I knew parasites were everywhere. After a leopard snatched my female cat, her kittens became quite ill. The one veterinarian in our region drove forty miles to see them, but he said that drugs were so scarce he couldn't give me any medication for my kittens. He needed to save the precious pills for the few hooved animals the farmers were able to raise in our tsetse fly–infested area. My kittens died agonizing deaths from parasite infections that I was helpless to treat. I wondered whether I would be lucky enough to avoid those deadly pathogens myself.

Boiling and filtering water and trying to remember to wash all fruit and vegetables in disinfectant, I survived the first year in good health. Into the second year, however, I became ill after eating a mango-and-papaya salad my cook had prepared with fruit from our own trees. Perhaps he had neglected to wash the fruit. Perhaps he had forgotten to wash his hands before working in my kitchen. I vomited green bile for days and staggered to the latrine hourly until there was nothing left. Weak and dehydrated, I lay on the veranda, too sick to care about anything. Even though I slowly recovered enough to go back to work, the dysentery continued. Other symptoms stayed with me. My eyes became clouded and bloodshot. Sharp, wrenching stomach pain doubled me over, and I was always fatigued.

Eating became extremely difficult. I knew my papaya trees produced fruit that soothed the stomach, so I began eating papaya every day. A friend suggested yogurt. That presented a problem, since I had not seen a cow anywhere in our region. When I finally managed to locate a farmer with a milk cow, I taught my cook to boil the milk on my two-ring gas stove, add the yogurt culture my friend gave me, and wrap the dish in a blanket. I had to buy a tiny propane-powered refrigerator, at the exorbitant price of two hundred dollars, to cool the yogurt. From then on, I lived on papaya, yogurt, and white rice. That was all I could keep down.

I felt better for a while, and then I became very ill again. I was hospitalized twice in Kampala, the capital city of Uganda. My British-trained Ugandan doctor said that he that thought I had amoebic dysentery, but the tests he ran didn't verify an amoebic presence in my system. Once, in an afternoon conversation over tea, I chatted with the Polish volunteer doctor in our village about health problems. He told me that the local people had the best skeletal health he had seen anywhere in the world. But they were so riddled with parasites, he said, that they were dying prematurely. He thought I had parasites, too, and he warned me that they could kill.

Over the next twenty years I lived in New York City, Istanbul, and Phoenix, but I never escaped the hovering shadow of my illness. As I continued to work as a teacher, my health problems persisted. Even though I ate natural foods, took no medications, rested, and exercised moderately, I didn't improve. I continued to consult physicians, none of whom had a diagnosis for me. Finally, in New York City at Columbia Presbyterian Hospital, I worked with a parasitologist who treated me for amoebic dysentery. The drugs he used to kill amoebic infections made me very ill while I was taking them. My health still did not improve. Later, living in Turkey, I became thinner and weaker and felt cold much of the time. Hospitalized once again, this time in Istanbul, I again received no positive laboratory test results. A Turkish pharmacist recommended chamomile tea. The pink tea was delicious with a dab of honey in it, and I felt slightly better when I drank it. During a stay in Tokyo, I was careful to eat no raw food because a Japanese physician there told me the Japanese can get parasites from eating raw seafood.

Then, in 1985, I had more bad news about my health. A gynecological exam found large fibroid uterine tumors that needed to be removed surgically. The gynecologist recommended a complete hysterectomy. I refused the surgery but agreed to a laparoscopy because of the doctor's concern that I might have ovarian cancer. Afterward, I didn't seem to recover from the anesthesia completely. From then on I felt groggy, disoriented, dizzy, and even more exhausted. Those symptoms continued until my frightening episode at the World's Fair in Vancouver.

During my 1986 hospital stay one tiny bit of hope glimmered. My husband took the test results from the hospital to a naturopathic physician. She was shocked at my low calcium level. She said she had seen only one lower test result, in an eighty-year-old woman hospitalized for osteoporosis. The hospital doctors had told me to ignore the calcium reading on that test. When I asked why I should ignore it, they said the test wasn't accurate. The naturopath disagreed and said I was in danger. In her opinion, my extreme weakness was the result of this low calcium level. At her suggestion, I began taking massive doses of calcium orally. Many weeks passed before I felt strong enough to walk again.

During that hospitalization, Steve and I had begun to realize that we would have to manage my survival and recovery ourselves, but we had little idea about how to proceed. My positive response to the naturopath's calcium supplement led me to a decision to search for alternative therapies that might help me recover from this dreadful mystery illness. My naturopath, a bright, compassionate woman who had graduated from a northwest naturopathic college, listened carefully to my symptoms. She then ordered blood tests and prescribed supplements and dietary modifications based on those results. That approach, she said, would improve my blood chemistry. In the months after my hospitalization, as I followed her directives, I didn't feel much better, but I was grateful that I wasn't growing worse. The success the naturopath was having in stabilizing my illness encouraged me to continue my search for gentle, nontoxic therapies that might assist my body in repairing itself. I continued to consult the naturopathic physician because she was helping me.

During those difficult times I was sustained by memories of my life in Africa. I had loved going on safari when I lived there. The most enjoyable trips for me were with friends from the Norwegian Peace Corps who were working as agricultural experts in the region of Uganda where I lived. We often headed north toward Atura and Gulu. One of us led our caravan driving a tough English Land Rover. The rest followed in battered Volkswagen Beetles roped with water tanks, gas cans, tents, food, beer, and even a concertina. The roads were tarmac, pressed red earth with a gravel finish. Bumping along with swirls of dust engulfing us, we relished a few free days away to explore this remote part of the planet. The lush, high savanna where we lived gave way to dry, barren plains. Only the occasional giraffe or wildebeest, well camouflaged, moved against the distant mountain backdrop.

One morning, as we jostled along, two of us spotted what looked like a clump of moving sagebrush. We signaled the caravan to stop. The sagebrush then stood up, transforming into three human beings. These were Karamojong tribesmen dressed in cloths the color of the earth tied at their shoulders. Decorated with mud-hair wigs draped with strings of colored beads, these men were tall, straight, and slender, with brilliant white teeth. We were surprised to learn we had been watched by human eyes. Crouching, they had been virtually invisible to us. I remember discovering a rather startling truth in our encounter with the Karamojong that day. I took it as a sign that I needed to pay more attention in my life. I needed to look closely and keep an open mind. Only then would I really "see" what was important for me.

While camping in Kabalega National Park, we often sat around a smoking campfire in the evenings, safe from mosquitoes and the threat of malaria for a time. With darkness, the animals of the plateau moved in closer. We saw their eyes reflecting the light as they circled behind our folding chairs. They seemed unafraid, perhaps because this place was so remote that the big-game hunters on safari didn't manage to find it before it became a protected area. I watched the animals, marveling at their beauty and stealth. Around the fire, my Norwegian friends sang folk songs to the sweet chords of their concertina. Listening to those melodies, watching falling stars cut swaths through the brilliant Milky Way, I was aware of being totally happy, perhaps for the first time in my life.

Another safari took us to Ngorongoro Crater, near Mount Kilimanjaro, in Tanzania. This is the crater floor of an inactive volcano accessed only along trails that the animal herds moving down from the Serengeti plains have made over the centuries. Swarms of elephants, rhinoceroses, buffalo, wildebeests, reedbuck, zebras, and Thomson's gazelles descend into the crater when it's too dry up on the plains for them to find food. The crater floor is lush with water and grasses where flocks of pink flamingos feed. The whole crater teems with life when the Masai tribesmen, who have grazing rights, move their herds of cattle through the wild animals. It seemed to me like a living Eden, with the animals eating and drinking peacefully in such close proximity to one another.

On these safaris I chopped wood, built fires, boiled water, set up tents, drove rutted roads, and walked long distances over rough terrain looking for wild game. Sometimes the heat nearly dropped us to our knees. A few times, we were charged by elephants. Once we were set upon by a rhino as we photographed from the Land Rover. His four tons missed our rear right fender by inches. Had he hit us, he would have flipped the vehicle and pummeled us to death. Twice we came upon poachers. My Norwegian friends shot their rifles to scare away these demons of the African savanna.

I felt a deepening sense of my own competence on these safaris. I was learning to cope with the African bush. I liked the toughness and determination that I was finding in myself. I enjoyed the adventure of it. I was beginning to feel that I could cope with most situations that presented themselves to me.

A few months into my illness, I began to think of the search for alternative healing for my illness as a safari. *Safari* is the Swahili word for *journey*. In East Africa, going on safari literally means leaving the comfort and safety of home. It signifies making one's way arduously through the wilderness looking for uncharted terrain, fresh oases of water and wild animals, pristine environments where life thrives. Now I was embarking on a metaphorical safari, seeking out timely information, traveling through unknown territories of learning, probing my own deep truths in order to get well. Stopping at each oasis of learning and experience, I would pitch a tent and take time to explore the truths I found there.

Steve helped me collect stacks of books and lists of phone numbers to begin my journey. When I felt I was ready, I embarked. The first book I opened was *Dr. Braly's Optimum Health Program,* by James Braly, M.D. Some of the information in that book, along with phone conversations I had with Dr. Braly in Los Angeles, put me firmly on the path toward alternative medicine. Although my vision was impaired, which made it difficult to read, and I had cognitive dysfunction, which made it difficult to understand what I was reading, I was determined to identify my illness and find a cure for it.

I knew that this safari would be difficult. I knew that it would take courage. I knew that I would be lonely as I passed through long stretches of parched desert searching for recovery. I also knew that I might find oases of alternative healing that could help me, if I was determined and careful about the types of therapies I used. Once I started the journey, for months at a time I found no help. Then, quite suddenly, my mirage of confusion would clear into a lush, warm, bright oasis of alternative healing that encouraged me to go on.

Over time, I gained more competence in researching my illness, talking to doctors, and managing my treatments. I was coping better with the illness, thinking more positively. I also was beginning to accept the possibility that I might not ever get well. I now knew that I might live with the illness for a very long time. Even though I didn't want to be sick any longer, I could tolerate it. I could make a life for myself even with these awful symptoms.

Five years into my healing journey, a medical doctor who was a specialist in environmental medicine finally ordered a new series of blood tests. One morning he called to tell me that I had systemic lupus erythematosus (SLE) with central nervous system involvement. The doctor explained that my immune system was attacking my own body. He also said that it was very serious and I might never recover. After searching so long for help, this was not what I wanted to hear. The doctor was angry that I had not been tested for lupus in 1986 when I was hospitalized and nearly died. The butterfly rash my doctors had ignored was, he said, an overt signal that I had lupus. I hung up the phone and sobbed.

After so many years on safari, however, I was organized and well equipped, and I had visited many healing oases. I was finding those oases by listening deeply to my body's messages, keeping an open mind, and trying not to be afraid. I visualized myself, sometimes parched with thirst, leading the caravan through swirling dusts of confusion, loneliness, and pain. I watched for any glimpse of enlightenment that stood up, like the Karamojong, and greeted me. Today, as I continue my journey, the Karamojong, with gentle smiles and soft words, sometimes shyly unbend and stand at full height in my mind. Then, reaching toward me, they offer the small painted gourds they carry with their spears. I have come to believe that those gourds are full of the learning and hope that have allowed my healing process to continue.

2

What Is Lupus?

For five years, I lived with a disease that went unnamed. This worried me, because I found it difficult to search for treatments when I did not know the nature of my illness beyond my obvious symptoms. On the other hand, I told myself there was a benefit to not knowing—as long as the illness did not have a name, it could not frighten me into believing there was no cure for it. Without a label, my illness had less power over me.

Five years after I became so desperately ill, I was told I had lupus. Finally hearing a name applied to my illness came as both a relief and a shock. It was a relief in the sense that I finally had a diagnosis to tell all the people who were impatient with me because my illness did not seem legitimate to them without a label. And it was a shock because I was told by my doctor that while I might get better—meaning that my lupus symptoms could go into remission—I would never completely regain my health.

When I heard the word *lupus* applied to my illness, I knew from my high school Latin that it meant *wolf*. Although I did not know why this illness had been named lupus, the metaphor seemed appropriate: a hungry, lean snout with sunken eyes staring quietly, wanting me, yet afraid to attack outright. Instead, this wolf hovered, paced, whimpered, growled, drooled, and waited, waited for his chance to move in for the kill. What an awful image, I thought. Because I love all animals, I tried to resist thinking of the wolf as my enemy, but I decided to let the metaphor stand since I couldn't think of a better one. The wolf's shadowy presence represented a more debilitating set of symptoms than I ever could have imagined. Now that I finally had a diagnosis, however, I determined to learn what I could about preventing the wolf's ravages.

The second thing I learned about lupus is that nearly four million Americans have it; that's more than have AIDS, cerebral palsy, multiple sclerosis, sickle-cell anemia, and cystic fibrosis combined. I also discovered how difficult lupus can be to diagnose accurately. Given my background, that came as no surprise. Systemic lupus erythematosus (SLE), commonly called lupus, is a chronic inflammatory disease that can go undiagnosed for years or can be misdiagnosed repeatedly. Even though researchers do not know how lupus is contracted, it appears not to be contagious. Lupus cannot be verified by simple blood tests. In fact, there is no single diagnostic test for lupus.

Many people with lupus find that their physicians ignore their symptoms of fatigue and general achiness, labeling them as having psychosomatic problems. Ninety percent of lupus patients are female. Our conventional medical system has a well-established history of dismissing female patterns of pain and fatigue as "hysterical" or "neurotic" and blaming the woman for her illness. It is probable, however, that even if medical incompetence and sexism did not exist, lupus often would go undiagnosed or misdiagnosed, because it is a disease that manifests in unpatterned, unusual ways. In an attempt to bring some clarity to the issue, in 1982 the American College of Rheumatology established a list of ten abnormalities that are specific to SLE. (See page 21.) In general, if a patient has experienced four or more of the abnormalities, not necessarily at the same time, she can be diagnosed with lupus. When my lupus tests were run, fully five years after I was in the depths of the illness, I had four of the ten criteria for lupus, all manifesting at once.

I wondered who my compatriots were. Who else out in the world had lupus? I was shocked to learn that lupus is more widespread than other more familiar diseases, such as multiple sclerosis and leukemia. It usually strikes women in their childbearing years between ages fifteen and forty; however, it can develop in young girls and postmenopausal women also. An infant can be born with neonatal lupus to a mother who has lupus. Mercifully, neonatal lupus usually disappears within six months.

Medical researchers are still perplexed about the origins of lupus, but it appears that a complex set of factors act in concert to cause lupus. Lupus occurs when a specific set of predisposing genes is exposed to a combination of factors, which could include environmental toxins, lupus-inducing drugs, infectious agents like bacteria or viruses, ultraviolet light, emotional stress, and physical trauma.

The presence of autoantibodies is pivotal for lupus. I wondered what autoantibodies were and searched sources to find out. A normal immune system produces substances called antibodies that fight the pathogens that cause disease. The specific purpose of these antibodies is to attack the invading pathogens, not our healthy tissue. In lupus, however, this marvelous immune response becomes hyperactive and begins assailing the body's own tissue. These "autoantibodies" may attack specific organs, such as the kidneys, or even other tissue, such as the bone marrow, limiting our red blood cell production and provoking severe anemia. Other autoantibodies may form immune complexes that produce inflammation in many of our tissues, such as muscles, connective tissue, heart, eyes, and brain. Not all lupus patients have high antibody levels, but even without antibodies they may have severe symptoms.

The question of whether our genetic makeup predisposes us to lupus is also pivotal to understanding why we get the disease. The genetic predisposition now appears to be well established. In February of 1997, researchers at the University of California at Los Angeles, who were funded by the National Institute of Arthritis and Musculoskeletal and Skin Diseases, announced that they had found the gene on chromosome 1 which renders people vulnerable to lupus.[1] The researchers believe that lupus is a genetically complex disorder and that it is likely that more than one gene determines whether a person will succumb to it. The researchers suggest that certain genes interact with each other and with triggers from the environment, like a virus or sunlight, to cause the disease. This breakthrough in lupus research should lead to blood tests for identifying persons susceptible to lupus. Those people could then be educated about many lifestyle changes that might help them avoid contracting the condition.

It is important to note that not everyone with the lupus gene gets lupus. A person who carries the gene probably will not contract lupus except in the presence of a number of other predisposing factors. Current research suggests that 10 percent of all people with lupus have a close family member who also has lupus. Only about 5 percent of children born to a parent with lupus will experience the disease. Research shows a higher rate of lupus among identical twins, probably because they have the same genes. Fraternal twins, who are no more genetically connected than ordinary siblings, have only a slightly higher risk of lupus than the general population. Can a person who is not carrying the gene get lupus? The most current genetic research indicates that only people with a genetic predisposition to lupus actually will come down with the disease.

A combination of two major factors can cause lupus. First, there may be immune complexes (conglomerates of antibodies, antigens, and viruses in the blood) that the body cannot break down. These complexes cause inflammation and destruction when they are deposited in tissues and organs. Second, lupus is elicited when one of the following immune responses occurs involving T cells and B cells, two subsets of lymphocytes: suppressor T CD8 cells are unable to subdue B-cell activity; or helper T CD4 cells may increase B-cell activity. Because B cells produce specific warrior chemicals called antibodies, this dysfunction of the suppressor T CD8 cells or helper T CD4 cells increases antibody levels, allowing the B cells to run amok, throwing the whole immune system out of balance. This in turn leads to the production of the dreaded autoantibodies. Research shows that when patients are ill with active lupus, they do not have normal levels of suppressor cells.[2]

What, I wondered, causes this problem with the suppressor cells? At present no one understands the very complex dynamics at work here, but it appears that lupus may stem from a complicated interaction of several factors, including specific environmental triggers and a genetic predisposition. One possible cause could be a yet unknown virus that moves into the body, deactivating the T lymphocytes. It is also possible that the female hormone estrogen is a major player in the pathogenesis of lupus. Several studies suggest that estrogen activates the immune system, while androgens (male hormones) somehow deactivate the immune response.[3] Blood tests have shown that I have autoantibodies to my own estrogen. I believe that this possible link between estrogen and lupus is intriguing and merits further research.

The following is a list of common lupus symptoms. It is illustrative of the agony most of us with lupus experience to varying degrees during active phases of our disease.

- **Fatigue:** This is the most universal and debilitating lupus symptom. It is much more than being tired; it is an exhaustion so deep that one sometimes can barely walk across a room. No amount of rest alleviates this kind of fatigue.
- **Pain:** Most of us with lupus feel as though we have the flu and arthritis at the same time. We experience generalized aching accompanied by severe pain at specific locations.
- **Rashes:** Lupus patients may have various kinds of rashes. The most common, however, is the butterfly rash, also called the malar rash. These rashes may burn, itch, and ooze if left untreated.
- **Hair loss:** Most of us see our hair thinning and find hunks of hair on our pillows and in the shower.
- **Fever:** Some of us run a low-grade fever of about 100 degrees all the time. I ran a low-grade fever constantly for more than three years. Others run a higher fever that may come and go. The fever may spike at night.
- **Sun sensitivity:** Most of us with lupus will experience rashes, fevers, or achiness after we are exposed to the sun.
- **Chest pain:** A sharp pain caused by inflammation of the lining of the heart and lungs is a typical lupus symptom.

- **Cold hands and feet:** Many of us feel that our hands and feet never get warm. About 20 percent of us have Raynaud's syndrome, in which our fingertips and toes turn a bluish color when exposed to cold.
- **Premenstrual flare-ups:** Many of our symptoms worsen just before our menstrual periods.
- **Dry eyes, dry mouth:** Many of us with lupus have Sjögren's syndrome, which occurs when autoantibodies attack the glands that produce saliva and the fluid that lubricates the eyes.
- **Easy bruising:** If the blood platelet count drops because the platelets are being attacked by autoantibodies, we will bruise more easily.
- **Edema:** This swelling around the eyes, ankles, or legs can be a sign of lupus and of kidney disease caused by the lupus.
- **Depression:** This can be severe, organic depression in which the lupus patient feels utterly helpless and hopeless.

Most of us with lupus have some or many of these symptoms, depending on the severity of the active disease. During my years with active lupus, I had all of these symptoms with the exception of easy bruising. I also had many other symptoms that are not on this list, such as heart palpitations, breathlessness, severe vision problems, difficulty hearing, and difficulty thinking logically.

The criteria that conventional medicine uses for diagnosing lupus are established through a series of complex blood analyses. Many of us are told that we meet at least four of the criteria, which means we have active systemic lupus erythematosus, but many other patients do not meet the criteria and are told they have only "lupus-like" disease. From my perspective, this is an academic distinction that has little merit in the context of overt lupus symptoms. Whether we are suffering from active lupus or "lupus-like" illness, it is imperative that we use all the self-care and alternative methods we can find to help our bodies heal.

What follows is a list of the ten criteria, the presence of four of which leads to a diagnosis of lupus. I am including a discussion of each criterion, because, in my opinion, many doctors do not offer enough information to lupus patients about these tests and what they indicate.

MALAR RASH

As many as half of all lupus patients experience this symptom. This rash usually appears as red, raised bumps across the cheeks and bridge of the nose. It may be a butterfly-shaped rash and may burn or itch or be hot to the touch. Although the precise cause of this rash is not known, it is likely aggravated by exposure to ultraviolet rays, since it appears on parts of the face that are exposed to the sun. Biopsies of these rashes illustrate that there are deposits of antibodies in the dermis, which is the deep layer of skin, as well as inflammation of blood vessels. This validates the presence of an autoimmune response. This rash can disappear spontaneously or with medical treatment and will not cause scarring.

DISCOID RASH

This rash affects about 25 percent of all lupus patients. It comprises round, scaly spots that appear on the ears, scalp, arms, or upper back. If left untreated, discoid rash can leave scars. It also can result in a form of hair loss called *scarring alopecia.* Like malar rash, it consists of inflamed cells, which indicate an autoimmune response.

PHOTOSENSITIVITY

Most lupus patients are photosensitive, that is, sensitive to the sun and other forms of light. Sun exposure may provoke a rash, fever, joint pain, fatigue, heart palpitations, and other symptoms of SLE. In some lupus patients sun exposure has even triggered kidney disease. Both ultraviolet A and B rays cause problems for lupus patients. Many of us are also sensitive to light from fluorescent bulbs (UVB) and even halogen lamps (UVA).

SEROSITIS

About half of all lupus patients have a painful inflammation of the delicate linings covering the abdominal cavity, heart, and lungs. This condition can be detected by chest radiography; electrocardiography, a noninvasive test that measures the heart's electrical activity; or echocardiography, a noninvasive test during which sound waves are bounced off the heart to provide a picture of it.

ARTHRITIS

Nearly all lupus patients have some form of arthritis that produces swelling and inflammation of the joints and ligaments in the hands, wrists, and toes. Many of us have arthritis in the larger joints as well. Arthritis usually worsens during periods of active disease and improves with periods of disease remission.

ORAL ULCERS

Possibly 40 percent of lupus patients have small lesions in the mouth that resemble cold sores. These are caused by inflammation and are usually painless.

NEUROLOGIC ABNORMALITIES

About 50 percent of lupus patients experience problems of the central nervous system (CNS). A wide range of disorders can result from involvement of the CNS in lupus. These conditions range from confusion and memory loss to acute epileptic episodes and psychosis manifesting as severe depression or schizophrenic symptoms, such as hallucinations and bizarre behavior.

RENAL DISORDER

Most SLE patients have some form of kidney abnormality. It can be mild, such as the leaking of protein into the urine, or severe, such as the breakdown of the kidney's ability to remove toxins from the blood. About half of lupus patients with kidney involvement suffer permanent kidney damage.

IMMUNOLOGIC ABNORMALITIES

When combined with other symptoms, four abnormalities in the blood can render a lupus diagnosis. The first is the presence of anti-DNA antibodies. Many lupus patients produce antibodies to their own DNA or genetic material. The second abnormality is the lupus erythematosus (LE) cell. The LE cell is found in the blood of 90 percent of patients with active SLE. It also is found, however, in patients with other autoimmune diseases, such as rheumatoid arthritis, scleroderma, and Sjögren's syndrome. Because this test is not specific to lupus, it is used rarely now as a diagnostic test for SLE. The third abnormal sign is the presence of antibodies to the antigen Sm. This is a highly specific test for SLE. If a patient tests positive for anti-Sm antibodies, he or she will very likely be diagnosed with SLE. The last abnormality is a false-positive serologic test result for syphilis. About 20 percent of SLE patients test positive for syphilis, even though lupus is totally unrelated to this or any other venereal disease. Some lupus patients generate antibodies that can be similar to those produced by patients trying to fight off syphilis; thus, the patient tests positive. In this circumstance, the attending doctor must be extremely careful to distinguish between these two diseases. If you have any one of the four preceding immunologic abnormalities, it counts as one point toward the four diagnostic criteria that constitute lupus.

HEMATOLOGIC ABNORMALITIES

These are four blood disorders that often are found in SLE patients. They are caused by autoantibodies that attack particular kinds of blood cells.

- **Hemolytic anemia:** Patients produce antibodies to their own red blood cells. If untreated, this condition can be very serious.
- **Thrombocytopenia:** Autoantibodies destroy the clotting cells, or platelets, in the spleen, which can lead to bleeding.
- **Leukopenia:** In this condition the leukocyte count is low, indicating that lupus is active.
- **Lymphocytopenia:** The count is low for lymphocytes (a subset of leukocytes), which impedes the body's ability to fight infection.

Any one of these four blood abnormalities counts as one point toward the four diagnostic criteria that combine to establish a diagnosis of lupus.

When I finally received my diagnosis of lupus, I had been on my safari into alternative therapies for nearly five years. With all the information I had found in many oases along the way, I was able to heal some of my symptoms successfully. As my journey continued, I found more help, which I will share with you in the following chapters.

Although I am ninety percent recovered from lupus now, I am still learning that enduring the barrenness, while being open to the adventure, is critically important. I also know that lupus, the wolf, may continue circling the campfire, watching me warily for the rest of my life. I may never be able to rid myself of his shadow, but I have learned that if I stoke the fire and create enough smoke, I can keep him at a distance. Ultimately, I am determined to send the wolf back into the mountains for good.

3

Your Liver

Each of us carries within us our own medicine.

Lakota tribal wisdom

Why Is the Liver Important?

I suspect that many of us with lupus have livers that were not functioning
well before we were diagnosed with the illness. We may have been born
with weakened livers. Our livers may have grown weak from infections,
such as hepatitis or mononucleosis. Also, as lupus patients, we may be taking pharmaceuticals that are toxic to our livers.

Could it be that a malfunctioning liver may even predispose us to lupus?
I believe this may be the case. When the liver is no longer able to cleanse the
blood of large protein molecules, our immune responses begin attacking
that protein, as they are programmed to do. Once our lymphocytes are in
this combative mode, with the continued presence of protein that is inade-
quately broken down, the white blood cells that normally protect us from
viral and bacterial invaders may begin attacking the protein in our own tissues. This aberrant activity of the immune system is called *autoimmune disease* in conventional medical terms. If the liver were able to filter the blood

properly, this chain reaction might not be set into motion, and we might not contract autoimmune conditions.

Quite early in my illness, I began to think that I had a problem in one of my organs. I ached everywhere; was puffy under my eyes, wrists, and ankles; and endured a constant, dull aching under my rib cage on the right side. I didn't think I had been engaged in any physical activity that could have cracked a rib. Through a process of elimination, I began to wonder whether my malady was centered in my liver, because that was the area of my body that hurt. I didn't know much about the liver except that I recalled having read that it had something to do with cleansing the blood. That led me to wonder not only about my liver but also about my blood. Was my liver able to bathe my blood? And what was the state of my blood? Was it clean and healthy or murky and weak? That led me to ponder a deeper question. Could the state of my blood be causing my illness? Conventional medicine defines lupus as an autoimmune disease. Today, after many years of reading and thinking about immune system malfunction, I think lupus could be defined more accurately as a blood disease. Early in my illness, I decided to follow my intuition about my liver and my blood. Learning all I could about them seemed an appropriate way to find ways to recover.

At this point, the safari I had planned through alternative healing took a change in course. Now my caravan and I trekked up and over great dunes of conventional medical books filled with pages of language about the liver and blood that was often impossible for me to understand. I became so confused and exhausted from the journey through those books that I was about to give up in frustration. Then my husband brought me a medical dictionary, which enabled me to decode some of the medical terminology. This allowed me to find the strength to try again to understand liver function and the blood's role in nourishing the body.

Gradually I arrived at an understanding of how the liver functions. Once I learned that toxins can weaken the liver, I kept reading. Then I learned that toxins actually can cause the liver to lose its ability to function efficiently, meaning that it is no longer able to cleanse the blood properly. This was information for which I had been searching, an oasis where I might

find the root of my illness. I pitched my tent, watered the camels, and set-
tled into my research. I was determined to persist with this difficult work,
because I knew that my illness was deep and life-threatening, and it was
clear to me that I would have to find my own path back to health. First I
needed to understand the liver's functions; then I would seek healing
approaches for my liver.

How Does Your Liver Work?

Found under your diaphragm just above your stomach, the liver is the
largest organ in your body. Thousands of chemical reactions take place in it
every second. Healthy livers deactivate hormones no longer needed, synthesize amino acids used in building tissues, and break proteins into sugar and
fat required for energy. The liver also produces lecithin, cholesterol, bile,
blood albumin vital to the removal of tissue wastes, prothrombin essential
to the clotting of blood, and innumerable enzymes and coenzymes.[1]

As the central chemical laboratory in the body, the liver is the storehouse
for all the alkaline elements needed for the body to stay healthy. After we
digest a meal, the blood from the intestines flows through the liver, entering through a large portal vein. At that point, the liver performs a number
of critical functions. As it filters the broken-down nutritional elements
from the blood, the liver synthesizes new body tissues, prepares fuel for oxidation and energy, and stores excess nourishment for future use. The liver
also neutralizes toxins and other harmful substances, eliminating them in
its excretion, which is called bile. Sometimes the power of the liver to neutralize these toxic substances is curtailed, however, because of insufficient
alkalinity in the body.[2]

With so many complex processes to complete, we may wonder how the
liver is ever able to function efficiently. The good news is that we have a
built-in system in our livers to protect us—the microsomal enzyme system,
or MES. This whole enzyme system helps deactivate and eliminate chemicals
such as hormones, pathogens in slightly spoiled foods, natural environmental toxins, and artificial chemicals. When the liver is healthy, the MES works
efficiently, giving us excellent protection from harmful substances.[3]

WHAT CAUSES STRESS TO THE LIVER?

The liver can be under great stress without our even knowing it. As lupus patients, we must be particularly vigilant about minimizing the stresses to which our livers are subjected. One of the most important things I learned about the liver is its dependence on sodium. Without enough sodium, the liver is stressed. As the most important alkaline element in the body, sodium is critical to the liver's ability to neutralize the acids in the body. When the liver is stressed by illness, environmental contaminants, or emotional reactions, however, it may lose much of its sodium. That sets off a chain reaction in which the liver loses its capacity to neutralize acids. At that point the weakened liver mistakenly releases toxic bile to the small intestine, which may provoke nausea. Even worse, this harmful substance is reabsorbed into the body. The resulting high acidity in the body then begins the cycle of illness.[4]

Those of us who succumb to the modern American diet, eating few fruits and vegetables and much overcooked meat, frequently have sodium-starved livers. How do we replenish and maintain the liver's sodium? Should we simply use the saltshaker more often? Definitely not. It's important to know that the liver needs *natural* sodium in order to keep the body in an alkaline state. We need to obtain sodium from carbon-based, organic sources, because the liver can metabolize organic sodium more easily than the inorganic compound sodium chloride, which is table salt.

Our need for sodium is only 500 to 1,000 mg a day, but many of us eat ten to fifty times more sodium than is considered necessary. Processed food in the United States is full of sodium chloride. Read the labels on canned foods when you're shopping, to gain an inkling of the out-of-control sodium in our canned foods. Even sweet foods like jams and soft drinks contain salt! This is not good for us. Excess table salt can cause serious health problems, such as hypertension. It also depletes the body's potassium. Low potassium, in turn, can contribute to life-threatening cardiac arrhythmias.

The richest source of natural sodium is nonstarchy vegetables, such as celery, zucchini, summer squash, crookneck squash, green beans, broccoli, cauliflower, brussels sprouts, radish, asparagus, cucumber, tomato, onion, leek, garlic, kohlrabi, and green, red, and yellow bell pepper. The second-richest source of natural sodium is lightly cooked liver and muscle meats (as opposed to nonliver organ meats such as tripe or sweetbreads). I believe we lupus patients need to eat more of these unprocessed foods to maintain our livers' natural sodium contents. As long as the liver has sufficient organic sodium along with a balance of the other electrolytes—calcium, magnesium, and potassium—it can keep us healthy by continuing to cleanse the blood properly.

In the early days of my illness, long before my lupus diagnosis, I often landed in emergency rooms with "panic attacks" and fainting spells. Laboratory tests run at those times showed nothing except that my potassium level was dangerously low. Although a doctor told me to begin taking potassium orally, he did not tell me about my sodium level. I now think that my sodium level was also low and that my liver function was impaired as a result. My liver most likely had struggled to clear the toxins from a general anesthetic I was given during the laparoscopic surgical procedure. It also had been attempting to mediate the toxins from two separate infections—one in my intestines, which I knew about, and the other, of which I was unaware, in my stomach. My liver undoubtedly was debilitated from carrying this load. I now think so-called panic attacks are the result of a severely stressed liver that is signaling the brain for help. When it receives the liver's SOS, the brain tries to protect us from everything that it perceives as a danger, causing the panic syndrome. From this perspective, it is possible that replenishing the liver's electrolytes—sodium, calcium, magnesium, and potassium—might stop the panic attack syndrome.

Another major stressor for the liver is environmental contamination. Pollution looms as a serious problem for all of us today. Chemical companies are pouring hundreds of new chemicals into the environment each year. Toxins in the food chain and the atmosphere are stressing us. Our systems are not able to recognize and process these "foreign" chemical compounds. Because living organisms adapt slowly, we may never be able to tolerate these chemicals. Meanwhile, the liver faces the burden of processing these contaminants before they can be neutralized and eliminated. It's no wonder our individual biochemical profiles may be disrupted, inducing poor health.

Many of us with lupus are sensitive to medications that can be toxic to our bodies. Our livers are stressed as they work at metabolizing the pharmaceuticals our doctors require us to take. Lupus patients aren't the only ones experiencing problems with pharmaceuticals, however. Five percent of hospital patients in the United States, or 1.9 million people, have significant adverse reactions to drugs administered by doctors. In fact, 2 to 4 percent of all hospital admissions—760,000 to 1.5 million people—are for reactions to doctor-prescribed drugs.[5] Medications may help us deal with the difficult symptoms of lupus, but we must be vigilant about how much medication we take. The more we take, the more we stress our livers.

Even our diets can burden us. The American diet has been shown to produce liver damage in rats. Highly refined carbohydrates, saturated fats, low protein and calcium levels, and high phosphorus levels all cause damage.[6] When we eat excessive amounts of fat and protein, we force the liver to work extremely hard to produce bile and other digestive enzymes. Moreover, the metabolic breakdown of protein creates harmful compounds, like ammonia, that can irritate or even be toxic to the liver.

When the liver is not functioning properly, we need to eat fewer fat- and protein-containing foods, such as meat and dairy products. And we should eat far more easily digested complex carbohydrates, such as rice and millet. These foods lessen the requirement for bile and therefore take a great load off the liver. Both Western and Eastern medicine teach that bile is a critically important bodily fluid that, when stagnant, causes sadness and disharmony. This condition is called *sluggish liver* in Western medicine and *liver stagnation* in traditional Chinese medicine.

How Does Traditional Chinese Medicine View the Liver?

The American health care system pays scant attention to the liver. While some conventional medical doctors do order liver tests, many of them seem to assign little importance to the liver. That leaves me concerned about those of us whose illnesses may be caused or aggravated by poorly functioning livers. Two conventional medical doctors have told me that they generally don't order blood tests for liver function. In their opinion, tests that show elevated liver enzymes can be difficult to interpret, in that they may not point to a definite diagnosis. Furthermore, these doctors say, liver tests cannot pick up subtle malfunctions of the liver. Only when a patient is clearly ill do they order a liver biopsy, which can pinpoint full-blown disease such as liver cancer.

Because Western medicine seems to de-emphasize liver health, I decided to research how other cultures view the liver. I was fortunate to find ancient wisdom in Chinese teachings about the liver that I have incorporated into my own healing process. A brief overview of the Chinese perception of the liver can provide us with a frame of reference for thinking about our own liver health. A primary belief in Chinese medicine is that the liver is the focal point of emotions. Traditional Chinese medicine, or TCM, holds that anger is associated with the liver and gallbladder. This tradition would say that someone who is chronically angry has an unhealthy liver or gallbladder. Conventional Western medicine does not connect wrath with the liver but says that the bile is storing excess hormones that a weak liver is not able to metabolize and eliminate.[7]

Although I had never considered myself an angry person, I was aware of feeling angry often during the worst years of my illness. This was a different sort of ire than I sometimes felt about being so ill. This emotion seemed to come out of nowhere, surprising me with its vehemence. It was unlike me, I thought, since I generally had been a fairly agreeable person. I was at a loss to identify the source of this rage, but discovering the Chinese medical model for anger suggested to me that I might have liver damage. It supported my suspicion that my liver function was impaired and needed healing.

The Chinese believe that the liver is the organ that regulates chi. We can define chi as the manifestation of all energy. Chi directs the whole activity of the body—the blood, the chi itself, and the healthy functioning of all the organs. The liver, says TCM, is particularly sensitive to anything that disrupts what the Chinese call its *free-and-easy wanderer* movement. Excessive emotions, for example, disrupt the flow of chi. When the energy in the liver is blocked, toxins build up that can cause cellular damage and poor functioning of our protective microsomal enzyme system (MES). When liver chi is disrupted, the resulting imbalance can produce a number of symptoms: emotional imbalance, rib pain or pressure, dizziness, headache, cramping, tendon problems, menstrual difficulties, jaundice, weak or blurry vision, and digestive disorders. I had all of these symptoms except jaundice.[8]

The liver, says TCM, is also susceptible to overstimulation. Alcohol, drugs, and too many spices (such as black pepper) can propel the liver into "blazing fire," or overactivity. This has a negative impact on the liver's enzyme production, causing heat to rise up to the head, with resultant headaches, facial flushing, thirst, dizziness, and ringing in the ears. I also had all of these symptoms during the worst years of my lupus.

TCM goes on to state that the liver regulates digestive activity. When the liver fails, we have digestive problems such as abdominal pain, nausea, burping, and diarrhea. In agreement with Western medicine, TCM teaches that liver function controls bile. If bile doesn't flow smoothly, it can lead to jaundice, loss of appetite, even a bitter taste in the mouth. Fats can't be tolerated well or assimilated, and the fat-soluble vitamins E, A, D, and K will not be well utilized. This situation can lead, in turn, to suppression of immune function. This complex condition can leave those of us with lupus, who often have suppressed immune responses, vulnerable to viral and bacterial infections. If we improve our liver function, however, we strengthen our immune response, thus protecting us against communicable disease.

TCM also tells us that a healthy liver oversees our emotions, harmonizing our feelings so that we live a well-balanced life. A strong, vibrant liver has a soothing effect, helping us maintain an even temper. When the liver is out of balance, however, our emotions become unbalanced, too, throwing the liver even more out of equilibrium and possibly worsening liver damage.

Finally, the Chinese tradition points out that the liver stores extra blood to be used when needed, such as during physical exercise. Imbalances occur if the liver does not have enough extra blood to store, which causes mouth and eye dryness—a condition that affects many of us with lupus. If the liver cannot store blood properly, it also leads to excessive menstrual bleeding.

Traditional Chinese practitioners check the fingernails for paleness or brittleness, which could mean that the liver is unable to nourish them properly. Since all of these aspects of liver functioning are synergistic, they are all interrelated. If you have many of the symptoms I've mentioned in the context of TCM, there is a strong likelihood that you have compromised liver function.

My research on the liver led me to the understanding that it is an extremely important organ, the purpose of which is to protect me. My next step was to learn how to care for my liver.

How Can You Nourish and Protect Your Liver?

The liver contains many filtering channels lined with special cells that engulf and break down foreign debris, bacteria, and toxic chemicals. But when the liver is burdened with toxins or bacteria, it can't perform its functions well and may even become damaged. In my search through alternative healing therapies, I found a startling statement about lupus in *The Encyclopedia of Natural Health*: "Gut-derived microbial toxins have been implicated in a wide variety of diseases including . . . lupus erythematosis." The authors go on to say that the liver and immune system are responsible for dealing with the toxic substances that are absorbed from the gut.[9]

Since I was quite certain that I still had an intestinal infection, these statements spoke directly to me. If my weakened liver could not neutralize the intestinal toxins, it could make me sick. Could there be a direct connection between my infection and what I thought was my impaired liver function? And could this have caused my lupus? Finding ways to restore my liver's health became even more imperative.

How can we nourish the liver's tone, to improve health? If we can maintain a balance between what the Chinese call the yin and yang—the soft and the hard—of our livers, that organ will stay quite healthy. One way to give the liver a rest so that it can restore balance is to detoxify. When we do this, chemicals break forth that may have been stored in our fatty tissue for years. The liver must be able to turn these fat-soluble chemicals into water-soluble compounds so that they move through the kidneys and out the bowels instead of being stored in the body. When the MES is healthy, the liver can perform these functions efficiently.

Try Gentle Detoxification Methods

What are some methods to detoxify and allow our livers to rest? Steve and I began searching for liver detoxification information early in my illness. One naturopath I was seeing used a diathermy machine that he placed on my liver for about thirty minutes per treatment. Diathermy works by applying heat to the affected area. After the treatment my whole body felt warm and tingly. I was always more relaxed, calmer, more content, and less achy after those treatments. My face also flushed, which suggested to me that my circulation improved. I believe that this treatment may help the liver's functioning return to normal. You may be able to find a naturopath or a chiropractor in your area who can treat your liver using a diathermy machine.

Simple self-care methods also can improve liver health. One way to encourage the liver to detoxify is to use a body brush. Body brushing stimulates the lymph system to flush toxins from the body. I bought a natural bristle, long-handled brush and followed suggestions in *The Colon Health Handbook*.[10] I have continued to brush my body for five minutes each day before I shower. Using the brush to stroke my limbs and trunk toward my heart stimulates my lymph system, enhancing my skin texture, my circulation, and my body's elimination processes.

Another approach to detoxifying and improving our liver health is to take saunas. In the fourth year of my illness we bought a Finnish sauna and installed it in our garage. A beautiful, small cedar room with a bench, it contains a simulated coal stove over which we pour water to create steam. Finnish people are aware of the health benefits of saunas. I grew up with Finnish friends who took saunas with their parents and grandparents. We non-Finns marveled at their radiant health—their flushed, robust color;

bright eyes; and soft, supple skin. Our sauna offers us a peaceful, restful place to detoxify our bodies. We enjoy using it at home rather than braving the crowds and high-priced memberships of health clubs.

One approach to liver detoxification that some American naturopaths use is hot castor oil packs placed over the liver. The origins of this home treatment reach back at least to early American colonial days. At the suggestion of a naturopath, I used a castor oil pack over my liver area for many months. It helped stop the aching in that part of my body, and I definitely gained energy. It's convenient to apply the oil pack at home when resting. To make a castor oil pack, soak a small cloth with castor oil, lay it over your liver, cover with a clean towel, and place a hot water bottle over it. Leave in place for thirty to sixty minutes.

Try Using Herbs

Because I have come to believe that lupus is a blood disease, I searched for a long time for ways to improve the quality of my blood. I learned that in natural healing, the liver is known as a blood-cleansing organism because it acts as a sort of "blood purifier." As I searched for ways to improve my liver's blood-purifying ability, I learned that the perspective in alternative health is that some herbs act directly to clean the blood, while other herbs help the liver clean the blood. Does this mean that these herbs literally "scrub" the blood? Not really. What happens is that the herbs stimulate blood flow through the liver, removing its congestion. They also protect liver cells and stimulate them to produce enzymes; in turn, this helps the body maintain a proper biochemical environment.[11]

By this time I knew that using herbs is a vital self-care approach to detoxifying the body and nourishing the liver. But which herbs could I try, and how should I use them? I didn't know. So I continued my research and discovered that herbal remedies are gaining popularity in the United States—$3.2 billion was spent on herbal products in 1997 alone.[12] There is a long tradition of herbal use in Asia, Russia, Europe, and South America. Because those cultures understand the importance of liver health, many of the herbs they use work specifically on the liver. I have incorporated a number of these herbs into my health regimen for recovering from lupus and have found each of them to be helpful. Before you decide to take any herbal product, however, be certain you inform yourself by talking to a naturopath or trained herbalist about the specific actions of the herbs and their possible side effects.

Naturopaths and herbalists use the herb called milk thistle, or Mary's thistle, to detoxify and tone the liver. It is native to southern Europe and Eurasia and has been used for many centuries to treat digestive and liver complaints. In modern German medicine it is widely prescribed as a phytomedicine (plant medicine) for liver disease. Milk thistle can be very effective but because many of us with lupus have food sensitivities, I urge caution. I took the capsules and felt worse, probably because I began to detoxify. I stayed with the regimen, however, and slowly began to feel much better, with less aching in my liver area and more energy. Be sure to try small quantities at first, to make certain you can tolerate it. Milk thistle is safe to take in small amounts.

Another excellent herb for helping the liver clean the blood is echinacea. It contains betaine, which has antiseptic properties and, with the caffeic acid glycoside in echinacea root, strengthens the enzyme pattern systems, or MES, in the liver. Echinacea also encourages the production of phagocytes, which clean wastes from the lymph, removing dangerous viral invaders from our bodies. This herb also helps clean and strengthen the kidneys, spleen, and pancreas. Its most important activity, for those of us with lupus, is its stimulation of the lymphatic system, which removes toxins from the blood.[13]

If you decide to try echinacea, you should not take it for long periods of time. Take it for only one week and then stop for a week. Later, extend the period that you take the herb to three weeks, with three weeks off, and so forth. Many healthy people I know take it only twice a year for two or three weeks as a toner for the immune system. If you feel yourself becoming sick with a cold or the flu, however, begin taking echinacea immediately.

Another wonderful way to purify the blood is by drinking rose hip or rose petal tea. The fruit, petals, and buds of roses contain huge amounts of vitamins A, B complex, C, D, E, P, and rutin. Imagine my delight at picking petals from the roses I grow organically, steeping them in a cup of boiling water, and knowing that, as I sip, I'm getting more vitamins than I would from ten to twelve dozen oranges! If you raise organic roses, pick some petals and brew up a pot of rose petal tea. If you have no fresh, chemical-free source of roses, talk to an herbalist about the quantity of dried rose hips to steep for tea. This is a pleasant way to help improve the health of your liver.

Another plant I only recently added to my herbal regimen is dandelion. It has been regarded highly as a liver remedy in folk medicine in China, Europe, India, and Russia and is thought to be indigenous to Tibet. The first written references to its use come from Arabian physicians of the tenth and eleventh centuries. In India, dandelion root has been cultivated and used for possibly thousands of years as a valuable liver and digestive remedy. Although it is considered a useless weed in this country, dandelion is high in nutritional value—higher, in fact, than most other vegetables.

Studies have shown that dandelion repairs liver function, thereby increasing the flow of bile. Last year we began picking the leaves from our own chemical-free organic dandelions, washing them thoroughly, and adding them to our salads. They impart a slightly pungent taste to the combination of greens. You can also steam dandelion greens and serve them as a side dish. Sipping a tea made from the leaves or taking an extract of dandelion root three times a day also will restore your liver's health. None of these methods of preparation destroys dandelion's ability to help your liver.

On my journey through TCM, I discovered tiny black pills called *hsaio yao wan*, which the Chinese traditionally have used to treat liver problems. The TCM doctor I was seeing was unable to explain to me in English the exact nature of this herb, but with some research I found that it is called bupleurum. This herb is a member of the parsley family, which commonly grows in grasslands in northern and central China and parts of Eurasia. The use of bupleurum appears to have very ancient origins and may even predate written language. The earliest records of the use of bupleurum in China are from the year A.D. 25.

Bupleurum is one of the best-known Chinese herbs for harmonizing liver function and protecting the liver against stress. It is used for unblocking liver congestion and dispersing stagnation. Bupleurum can help alleviate such symptoms as dizziness, vertigo, emotional excesses, and menstrual problems. It also can relieve bloating, nausea, and indigestion. I have found that it has reduced all of these symptoms for me. And it has a mildly calming effect. You can find hsaio yao wan pills wherever Chinese herbal formulas are sold. It comes in an amber glass bottle in a green and white box that is clearly marked. My Chinese doctor has told me that it is the "number one" prescribed herbal formula in China. I take six of the tiny black pills three times a day. It is inexpensive and safe to use.

Use Dietary Supplements to Nourish Your Liver

In addition to herbs, there are a number of other nutrients I have found that can help support the liver. These nutrients can be of great benefit to those of us with lupus in assisting our livers to break down toxins. I have added all these nutrients to my diet, either as food or in capsule form, and I believe they have contributed greatly to my recovery.

If I could take only one vitamin, it would be vitamin C. In my opinion, it is a "wonder vitamin." When taken in generous amounts, vitamin C can protect the liver, even from highly toxic substances. While it improves nearly all bodily functions, it plays specific roles that help lupus patients. First, it is needed for the formation of collagen, a protein connective tissue that holds the cells together. Lupus is sometimes called a *connective tissue disease*, because the collagen breaks down. Second, vitamin C is needed for the creation of the prostaglandins PGE_1 and PGE_3, which reduce pain. This vitamin is also a powerful antioxidant, detoxifying many harmful free-radical substances in the body. Finally, vitamin C is profoundly effective in strengthening the immune system. It aids in the production of interferon, the body's own antiviral agent. It also stimulates the phagocytes—the body's white blood cells, which fight infection—to devour viruses and bacteria.[14]

I have taken 10 g (10,000 mg) of vitamin C a day for many years, because I feel that I need the antioxidant protection it gives me. We can obtain vitamin C from food sources, such as citrus fruits, rose hips tea, broccoli, spinach, chard, kale, peppers, strawberries, currants, brussels sprouts, and cauliflower. In addition to eating many of those foods, I have chosen to supplement vitamin C in powdered or crystal form, to raise my blood serum level of vitamin C. Taking buffered vitamin C is best, because it is nonacidic, thereby minimizing damage to tooth enamel and gastrointestinal irritation.

Vitamin A also can protect the liver against toxic drugs and chemicals. It is very important for healthy mucous membranes and healthy skin. Like vitamin C, vitamin A can be helpful for lupus patients in its antioxidant role, controlling highly destructive free radicals. Vitamin A strengthens the thymus gland, the master gland of the immune system. Very important, too, in the alleviation of lupus symptoms is vitamin A's ability to prevent release of excessive inflammatory prostaglandin (PGE_2). That means it may help lower pain level. Vitamin A can help those of us with lupus in another important way. We know that sunlight can increase our lupus symptoms. Vitamin A has the ability to act as an internal sunscreen against the damaging effects of ultraviolet rays from the sun.

Another helpful nutrient for those of us with lupus is beta-carotene, which is closely associated with vitamin A. In the past, it was thought of merely as a precursor to the formation of vitamin A. Now, however, a number of independent functions have been discovered. It has emerged as a potent antioxidant, blocking destructive free radicals. Like vitamin A, beta-carotene helps prevent inflammation, may lower pain level, and also acts as an internal sunscreen.

Perhaps beta-carotene's greatest promise lies in cancer prevention. A documented study in the 1980s proved that it can protect body tissue from vitamin A depletion. This was associated with lower lung cancer rates among both smokers and nonsmokers. Another study also documented significant antitumor effects in people taking beta-carotene.[15]

We can obtain vitamin A by eating fish or animals that naturally produce the nutrient in their bodies. The best sources of beta-carotene are papaya, sweet potatoes, spinach, collard greens, cantaloupe, and carrots, particularly carrot juice. Other good sources of beta-carotene include squash, kale, turnips, beet greens, mango, dried apricots, broccoli, tomatoes, and asparagus. When our livers are functioning properly, they can convert the beta-carotene in vegetables to vitamin A, so that we obtain sufficient quantities of both of these helpful vitamins through the foods we eat.

Even though I eat many foods that contain vitamin A and beta-carotene, I also supplement my diet with each of these nutrients. I take a standard dose of vitamin A at 25,000 IU and a standard dose of beta carotene at 20,000 IU per day. Vitamin A is very safe at that level, but be aware that toxic levels are reached at doses of 100,000 to 300,000 daily over several weeks. Beta-carotene is also safe at the standard dose but will cause yellowing of the skin if taken in excess. That effect will disappear upon lowering your beta-carotene intake.[16]

Vitamin E is another excellent source of protection for the liver. When taken in liberal amounts, it has been shown to prevent development of scar tissue in the liver caused by injury from industrial chemicals. It protects vitamin C from oxidation. It also enhances the efficiency of the muscles—especially the heart muscle—by reducing its oxygen needs. Because my particular form of lupus has caused my immune system to attack my heart muscle, I have felt vitamin E is critically important in protecting my heart. Many of us with lupus have antibodies to our own DNA. Vitamin E protects our genetic material from free-radical damage.[17] This vitamin can offer pain relief as well; one medical study in Israel in the 1980s found that vitamin E can provide significant pain relief to arthritis sufferers—particularly for osteoarthritis.

Vitamin E can bolster immune strength, which is very important for lupus patients. This means that it can help quell viral and bacterial infections. Vitamin E holds promise for treating cancer, heart disease, allergies, aging, and wound healing. Conclusive tests conducted in the 1980s showed that vitamin E has a positive effect on autoimmune diseases—specifically SLE.[18] Good dietary sources of vitamin E are wheat germ oil, nuts, seeds, whole grains, rice bran, and soybeans. You can take supplements of Vitamin E in capsule form; 50 to 1,200 IU per day is a safe amount. When

I began taking vitamin E, I reacted to it with heart palpitations, dizziness, nausea, and problems with my eyesight. If this happens to you, try the dry form of vitamin E. You may be reacting to the oil in the vitamin E preparation rather than the vitamin E itself.[19]

There are a number of amino acids that I have found very helpful in minimizing my lupus symptoms. Methionine, for example, is necessary for the proper function of the liver, gallbladder, and kidneys. It helps the liver convert toxic substances to water-soluble compounds, which are then excreted through the kidneys. This action helps protect the liver from toxic damage, which is important for those of us taking medications. Methionine is a building block for other important amino acids.[20]

Choline also can benefit the liver. Strictly speaking, it is not a vitamin but is synthesized in the body from the amino acids methionine and serine. The strength of our cell membranes depends on choline. It is also critical in the transmission of nerve impulses and in memory. It is important to the regulation of fats and cholesterol, and it assists the liver in breaking down those nutrients. An average supplemental dose of choline would be 300 to 1,000 mg a day. Doses larger than 2,000 mg can provoke diarrhea. You can obtain choline in your diet by eating egg yolk, animal liver, and all dried beans.

Another amino acid, L-carnitine, is manufactured in the body from two other amino acids, lysine and methionine. L-carnitine can help the liver handle alcohol consumption, a high-fat diet, and chemical exposure. It aids the liver in converting fatty acid loads. It also serves as an efficient transporter of fatty acids through the cell membranes into the energy creation center of the cell, the mitochondrion. I believe those of us with lupus have cells that are underoxygenated. This may be one of the reasons we often experience such deep fatigue. L-carnitine has the potential to help our livers give us more energy. I take a low to average dose of L-carnitine of 1,000 mg a day. There are no vegetable sources of L-carnitine; food sources are mainly muscle and organ meats.[21]

In my opinion, selenium is vital for lupus patients. Unfortunately, it is relatively difficult to obtain in our diets. It's important to know that a selenium deficiency can damage the liver. There is widespread selenium deficiency in this country. Because much US soil is selenium deficient, food crops grown in those soils also will be deficient, and people who eat those crops will be lacking in sufficient selenium. Selenium acts synergistically with vitamin E, working as a major antioxidant to protect against damage to the cell membranes and to the RNA/DNA genetic material. It influences the healthy functioning of the immune system and the liver. It also strengthens the retina of the eye and helps prevent cataracts. When we are deficient in selenium, we may find brown spots on our skin, have poor hair and skin tone, suffer repeated infections, or have heart disease or cataracts.

You can obtain selenium from onions, milk, eggs, kelp, garlic, mushrooms, organically grown foods, seafood, most vegetables, and brewer's yeast. I take it in supplement form to guarantee that I am getting enough of this important nutrient. A dose of 50 to 400 μg a day is sufficient. Selenium needs to be taken with vitamin E in order to work efficiently.[22]

CAN THE LIVER RECOVER?

After all my research on the liver, I was pleased to learn that even if the liver has been damaged by alcohol, infection, medications, or nutritional deficiency, it can recover quickly. Unlike the brain or the heart, the liver can heal itself with encouragement. Dr. Andrew Weil states in *Spontaneous Healing* that he is impressed with "the ability of the liver—the largest organ in the body and one of the most active—to regenerate lost tissue. You can cut away most of the liver—up to eighty percent of it—and the remaining portion will restore the lost substance in a matter of hours, as long as the tissue is normal."[23] This is very good news for all of us with compromised liver function.

My early journey through alternative health literature taught me many approaches to restoring the liver's vitality. I had learned about self-care methods, herbs, and supplements for the liver. I did not use all the approaches at once, because I was discovering them over a period of months to years. My research led to many new ideas, which I formed into a daily regimen for treating my liver. Carefully following that protocol each day began to help me feel better. My energy level slowly recovered, my pain level began to diminish a bit, and my digestion improved. I had made a good start at restoring my health. But I knew there was much more unknown territory to explore. With a higher energy level, I decided to continue my safari. This time I would search for a new oasis, one where I could learn about the best foods to eat for recovering from lupus.

4

Your Diet

Food is your best medicine.

Henry G. Bieler, M.D.

How can we help our bodies recover from lupus and regain their natural vibrancy? Could something as simple as food be the answer? When I read Dr. Bieler's quote in 1986, I was skeptical about the possibility that my diet could heal me. But since I had promised myself to explore all options for regaining my health, I decided to keep an open mind. Loading my traveling gear and harnessing my camels once again, I resumed my journey through alternative health care searching for information on nourishing diets.

After reading many books on nutrition and talking with a number of nutritionists, however, I realized that no one really knew what I should eat for recovery from lupus. Some sources said I should eat no animal protein, some that I should eat a diet low in protein, and others that I should eat a great deal of protein. None of the experts were voicing concern about the effects of refined sugar on chronically ill people, when I knew from experience that eating sugar made me feel worse. Slogging through the food controversies suggested to me that I was going to have to find my own way out of the dietary maze. I began, through trial and error, to find a way to eat to alleviate my symptoms.

For more than twelve years now I have practiced the specific guidelines to healthy eating that I created for myself. Although conventional medical doctors generally do not stress diet in their treatment of lupus patients, I believe dietary changes can be pivotal in mitigating lupus symptoms. Diet is particularly important when we are experiencing flare-ups of disease activity. By eating simple, nourishing food that the body can absorb easily and the liver can put through chemical conversion and filtering processes, we may be able to move through a lupus flare-up with less agony. Adhering to that same nourishing diet over time can help rebuild our bodies to the point where we may regain some of the vitality we had before lupus entered our lives.

On my safari into nutritious eating, a particularly arduous stretch of desert appeared when I was hospitalized. The institutional food was awful. The meat was overcooked and tough, the fish was fried, the potatoes were a white tasteless glob, the white rice was barely cooked, and the vegetables had been boiled nearly to paste. There was no salad other than Jell-O, and I had not seen fresh fruit or fresh vegetables on my plate in the four days that I'd been hospitalized. Meal after meal, the institutional food sat on the plate, full of fat, salt, and preservatives; soft and colorless; lacking in fiber; daring me to eat it. Before my hospitalization, I had lost thirty pounds in four months. Even though I had been trying to eat as much as I could, I was continuing to lose weight and growing weaker. My physical appearance alarmed my family. "Sharon," they said, "you must eat."

The hospital meals were the last straw. I simply could not eat them. By that time I was often feeling frantically hungry. We asked for better food, such as baked, poached, or broiled meat or fish; complex carbohydrates such as brown rice, bulgur, or whole wheat pasta; and fresh salads, but none of our requests were filled. We wondered what we could do. I recalled that in countries where I had lived, such as Uganda and Turkey, families brought food in for their relatives who were hospitalized because the hospitals could not finance meal preparation. Might we do the same thing? In a flash of empowerment, my parents and my husband decided that they could indeed bring me home-cooked meals.

Imagine my relief when that delicious organic brown rice, steamed fish, organic salad, organic nuts, and filtered water arrived every evening. I can remember tentatively beginning to eat the healthy food, praying that it would keep me alive. And it did. After a few meals, my nausea began to subside. I finally began to feel full and was able to sleep. Dr. Bieler's words held a particular irony for me at that time. "Food is your best medicine." The hospital food was my worst medicine, but the nutritious food brought in to me by my family proved to be my best medicine during that period of deep illness.

Over subsequent weeks, after I left the hospital, I continued to eat that simple diet and felt somewhat better. Whenever I deviated from that narrow combination of organic foods, however, I grew dizzy, weaker, and more confused. What could be causing those symptoms? I suspected I had food allergies. The naturopath agreed and suggested we run food allergy tests. Called Immunoglobulin G radioallergosorbent tests (IgG RAST), these assays measure blood antibodies to food antigens. When the number of antibodies is higher than normal, it means that the immune system is attacking protein molecules of that particular food in the bloodstream. This leads to the production of histamine, which is one of the chemicals that makes us feel ill during allergic reactions.

My IgG RASTs verified several food allergies. The naturopath also suspected that I was reacting to nonfood compounds that IgG RASTs do not test for, such as chlorine, nickel, mercury, tin, lead, formaldehyde, printer's ink, and diesel fumes. I consulted a kinesiologist and found, through muscle testing, that I seemed to be reacting to nickel, diesel fumes, vitamin E, ascorbic acid, and even the smell of cooked cabbage, which contains sulfur compounds.

The underlying question was what was causing all these sensitivities? I now think that my immune response was fighting so hard to kill the two infections in my body (a stomach infection and an intestinal infection) that it had begun randomly attacking other protein molecules in my blood. This is the classic allergy pattern. I believe that another contributing factor was that my liver was under so much stress from the toxins of the infections that it was not able to convert and release the environmental toxins to which I was being exposed.

I wondered what I could do, if anything, to ameliorate those allergic reactions. Restricting my diet and avoiding metals and chemicals as much as possible seemed to be the only approach available. Even though we did not know then that I had lupus, in retrospect I think it's possible that many lupus patients have food and chemical sensitivities that contribute to the illness. It's important, therefore, for each of us to eat as healthily as possible.

COMMITTING TO EATING NOURISHING FOOD

What can you do to create a diet for yourself that will minimize liver stress and lessen your lupus symptoms? First, pay attention to your body to discover what foods it can and cannot tolerate. Do you suspect you have food and chemical sensitivities? If so, take the IgG RAST. They are an efficient way of finding allergies that may be contributing to the toxic load your body is struggling with during the times when lupus is active. Then do everything you can to avoid the substances to which you are allergic.

Books and articles on nutrition also will provide you with ideas for improving your diet. If you are too ill to read, ask a friend to read the information for you and then give you a summary. In addition to reading, you might consult a certified nutritionist who has studied at a naturopathic college. Finally, TCM could be a resource for you, since the Chinese have been aware of healing foods for thousands of years.

Dr. Bieler offered me assistance with my questions about the best foods to eat. A brilliant, now deceased, physician who used nutritional approaches to help his patients recover from illness, Dr. Bieler wrote an excellent book in the 1950s entitled *Food Is Your Best Medicine*. In his book, Dr. Bieler explains that the ancient Greek physician Hippocrates, the father of modern Western medicine, taught his patients what to eat to cure themselves. Since I have tried to listen closely to ancient wisdom, this idea was a wake-up call for me.

Hippocrates was probably not the first healer to look upon food as medicine. In fact, the knowledge that we can heal ourselves with certain foods may be hundreds of thousands of years old. There is even evidence that wild animals know which foods to eat to feel better. Dr. Jane Goodall, an anthropologist, found that the chimpanzees she observed over a period of more than twenty years near Gombe, Tanzania, ate certain leaves when they were ill. Subsequent tests of those leaves verified that the plants contained phytochemicals that had antiviral and antibacterial properties. Certainly, paying attention to what we eat may help us get well. In an age when pharmaceuticals have gained such prominence, heeding Hippocrates' learned ideas about food can offer us another approach to healing.

HEALING WITH ALKALINE FOODS

If we are to get well and stay well, it's critical that there be a proper ratio between acid and alkaline foods in our diets. The natural ratio in a normal, healthy body is four parts alkaline to one part acid, or 80 percent to 20 percent. In America, our diets are often 20 percent alkaline to 80 percent acid. When we are ill, our bodies become more acidic from the toxins of the infection, which means that during illness we need to stress alkaline foods even more. When we maintain the 80 percent alkaline to 20 percent acid balance, we can generally resist disease more effectively.

You can start improving your body's alkalinity by eating vegetable broth you prepare at home. Vegetable broth is one of the standard beverages in all biological healing clinics in Sweden. Recovering patients there always start the day with a big mug of vegetable broth—a cleansing, alkalinizing, and mineral-rich drink.[1] This broth can help those of us with lupus, because it replenishes the electrolytes our livers need to function properly.

Years ago I began preparing a delicious drink called Bieler's broth, a combination of lightly cooked green beans, celery, zucchini, and parsley that I found in Dr. Bieler's book. It is a soup rich in sodium and potassium that is excellent for nourishing and resting the liver. It also can help the pancreas control the level of blood glucose.[2] An added benefit of the broth is that it restores the body's alkalinity. According to Dr. Bieler, even one correct meal assists a toxin-saturated body to regain balance.

To make Bieler's broth, steam two medium zucchini, a handful of green beans, and two stalks of celery until they are very soft; reserve the water used for steaming the vegetables. Place the vegetables and one to two cups of the reserved water in the blender and blend for one to two minutes until smooth. Add fresh parsley and serve hot. Store in the refrigerator no longer than two days; then prepare a new broth. Steaming vegetables avoids the overcooking that destroys the enzymes and vitamins that are vital to the body.

Here is another tasty vegetable soup recipe that provides sodium and potassium and has a high alkaline content. Even though it is not quite as easy for the body to digest as Bieler's broth, it can add variety to your meals. In a large saucepan, sauté diced celery, carrot, zucchini, broccoli, cauliflower, cabbage, onion, and garlic in a little pure water. Then cover with water and add one tablespoon of oregano, one tablespoon basil, and a bit of salt. Simmer half an hour and serve. You can add diced new red potatoes or sweet potatoes for variety.

One of the best alkalinizing and mineral-rich dishes I make is a vegetable broth from Paavo Airola's book *How to Get Well*. Combine two large, chopped potatoes (half-inch pieces), one cup sliced or shredded carrots, one cup chopped or shredded celery, one cup of your choice of beet tops, turnip tops, parsley, and the like. Add garlic, onions, and/or natural herbs and spices. Put all the vegetables into a stainless steel utensil, add one and a half quarts of water, cover, and cook slowly for about half an hour. Strain, cool until just warm, and serve. If you don't use the soup immediately, keep it in the refrigerator and warm it up before serving.

In addition to cooked vegetables, we also should eat raw vegetables. They are important to us as a source of roughage, and they keep the contents of our intestines from becoming too dry. But when we're ill, we need to be careful of how many raw foods we eat, because they're difficult to digest. When we're feeling better, we can increase the number of colorful vegetables in our diets. The high levels of antioxidants in the most brightly colored vegetables help reduce the free radicals that contribute to our illness.

It is a better idea to juice raw vegetables than to eat mounds of them when we're ill. This "natural water" from the juice is a kind of water the body needs.[3] A number of doctors have found the healing properties of fresh juices to be remarkable. Max Gerson, M.D., watched many of his cancer patients recover on the juice therapies he recommended as part of a larger curative regime. The late Max Bircher-Benner, M.D., who ran a famous health clinic in Europe, believed that green juices were the most therapeutic treatment available for healing deep illness.[4]

An excellent juice for those of us with lupus is a raw potassium drink. It is invaluable at helping people heal, because it provides a source of easily assimilated vitamins, minerals, and enzymes. A good recipe for live potassium juice comes from Norman Walker's book *Fresh Vegetables and Fruit Juices*. You can make one pint of this healthful drink by combining seven ounces of carrot juice, four ounces of celery juice, two ounces of parsley juice, and three ounces of spinach juice.

From my reading in nutrition, I learned that vegetable juice provides not only alkalinity but also active enzymes that help the liver filter chemicals and make chemical conversions. Juice sounded like such a good idea that I bought a juicer and began drinking a glass of fresh vegetable juice each day. After some weeks on this regimen, I realized that if I missed the juice for a few days I did not feel as well. I had less energy and was more depressed. It seemed reasonable to keep drinking vegetable juice.

The nutritionists Cherie Calbom and Maureen Keane, in *Juicing for Life* offer an excellent short course on the benefits of eating raw food and drinking raw juices. They state that a diet high in raw foods can reverse the bodily degeneration that accompanies long-term illness and help improve energy and emotional balance.[5] Be aware, however, that excess carrot juice can turn your skin yellow. Green juices, if taken in very large quantities, can irritate an inflamed intestinal lining. One glass of fresh vegetable juice a day is sufficient to increase alkalinity and improve your health.

When we are eating these rejuvenating diets and trying to rebuild our bodies, we may experience a "physiological housecleaning" as our bodies begin to excrete toxins from our tissues. Many of us with active lupus already endure varying degrees of mental confusion, aching joints, muscle and joint stiffness, headache, nausea, vertigo, and stomach or intestinal upset. As we begin to lose toxins, we are likely to have withdrawal symptoms, such as fatigue, racing pulse, dizziness, more aching in the joints, and more headaches. I endured all of these discomforts because I was trying so hard to get well. Once I made it through the first few days of the detoxification process, I felt much better.

Many alternative health regimens suggest fasting as a way to regain health. I avoided fasting for a long time for two reasons. First, because I was generally weak from the effects of lupus, I felt that I needed to eat lots of solid food. Second, I love good food and dreaded giving it up, even for a short time. When I finally decided to try fasting, I ate no food and drank only juice for four days, but I became weaker, dizzier, and extremely thirsty. I realize that I was most likely going through detoxification, but I felt that it was too much for a body to endure that was already wracked by lupus symptoms. I do not think those of us with lupus should fast. It is too radical a dietary approach for us.

FEELING BETTER WITH COMPLEX CARBOHYDRATES

In the early days of my illness I was dizzy and hungry, often only a half hour after I had eaten. I suspected that I had blood glucose problems that were causing those symptoms. By doing more research I learned that foods that move through the system quickly and hit the bloodstream fast raise insulin levels. This high insulin level is not good for us—it makes us vulnerable to diabetes. I learned that I needed to eat foods that digest more slowly, to keep my insulin levels lower and more constant. I therefore stopped eating all forms of sugar, all baked goods, and white bread. Instead, I began substituting more complex carbohydrates, such as whole grains and the few legumes I could tolerate. The vegetables in the broths I was eating added complex carbohydrates to my diet.

Consulting with a Vietnamese physician who had immigrated to this country, I learned that brown rice and brown rice gruel are life-sustaining. He told me stories of starving Vietnamese peasants brought to his hospital who, unable to eat and on the verge of death, began to respond when nurses fed them brown rice gruel. In his opinion, brown rice is a miracle food. He says brown rice is particularly helpful for Americans because we, as Westerners, have not eaten it for centuries as a staple, as many Asians have, and thus have not developed allergies to it.

This doctor's stories encouraged me to purchase a twenty-pound bag of organic brown rice at our local food co-op. Since then, our family has eaten brown rice four to seven times a week for the past ten years. We rarely eat white rice, because it is primarily starch and contains few nutrients. The bran and husks of brown rice, however, contain protein, B vitamins, and fiber. For many years now I have been combining brown rice, lentils, legumes like pinto beans, large amounts of vegetables, and small portions of animal protein. This diet has helped me to feel better. Root vegetables supply complex carbohydrates as well, but according to Steven Masley, M.D., Americans eat too many root vegetables, particularly potatoes, which raise the blood glucose levels. We should avoid them or eat fewer of them and substitute pasta, lentils, and whole grain bread instead, which keep the blood glucose levels more stable.[6]

Other grains that supply complex carbohydrates and do not produce surges in blood glucose include whole grain pasta, amaranth, barley, bulgur, and buckwheat. Many legumes are also excellent sources of complex carbohydrates, helping to keep the blood glucose stable. Even though lupus patients may be unable to eat some legumes, you might find that you can tolerate other legume varieties. It's worth experimenting to see which legumes you are able to eat. The best blood glucose stabilizers in the legume family are lentils, peanuts, and soybeans. Other good legumes for balancing the blood glucose are kidney beans, chickpeas, green peas, and pinto beans.

To increase my fiber intake and to move digested food more quickly through my system, I also began taking one to two tablespoons of psyllium husk per day. In addition, because I have stomach irritation, I make a gruel from slippery elm that coats the mucosal lining of my stomach and intestines, aiding digestion and elimination. Uncooked fruits and vegetables add fiber, too. It's important that we "bulk up" on whole, alkaline foods, so that we are less tempted to eat sugar and other acidic foods. Generally, you can find psyllium husk at health food stores and slippery elm powder where bulk herbs are sold.

Considering a Vegetarian Diet

The question of whether lupus patients should eat a strictly vegetarian diet is difficult to answer. The naturopaths I consult do not recommend vegetarianism, because they believe the body needs some animal protein to function properly and remain strong. Even though the herbalist Christopher Hobbs was a vegetarian for twenty-one years, he now thinks it's important to eat fish two to three times a week or even as seldom as once every ten days.[7]

From my research findings, I decided that I had been eating too much meat. For this reason, during the first two years of my illness, I ate large portions of grains and vegetables, no dairy, and only small amounts of fish and chicken. That was essentially a macrobiotic diet, though I did not know it at the time. I learned later that a macrobiotic diet is nonmucus forming, low in fat, high in vegetable protein and fiber, and very alkalinizing.[8] The diet that I had created for myself helped my digestion and kept me feeling full, but I was unable to gain any weight, which was a primary problem during my active bouts of lupus. My physical weakness continued. Later, I returned to eating more animal protein but continued to avoid red meat. Some vegetarians I have known say they became weak over time, but others claim they have always remained strong. No one seems to understand fully the dynamics of vegetarianism yet, and it is still the subject of controversy.

Andrew Weil is a medical doctor who often uses unorthodox methods. He believes health is tied to diet, and in his book, *Natural Health, Natural Medicine,* he makes a specific dietary suggestion for lupus patients. Weil states that high-protein diets can irritate the immune system, aggravating allergies and autoimmune disease.[9] In view of that, he suggests that those of us with lupus cut back on animal protein. Calling lupus a "protein disease," he hypothesizes that the less protein we ingest, the less our hyperactive immune systems will attack protein in our tissues and organs in our bodies. Weil thinks lupus patients should eat very little protein—only 10 percent of our daily diet.

It is important for us to eat plant protein, however. Legumes are a good source of protein but are difficult to digest. Many of us with lupus have legume sensitivities. Grains also contain some protein. One way to cut down on both animal protein and legume protein is to eat a simple, plant protein diet for a time to give the body a rest. This diet consists of cooked cereals for breakfast, plain salads for lunch, and cooked, nonstarchy vegetables for dinner. My legume sensitivity has precluded me from becoming a vegetarian, because I cannot substitute beans for animal protein. If you aren't sensitive to legumes, however, vegetarianism could be a wise choice for you, according to Daniel Wallace, M.D., author of *The Lupus Book*. He agrees with Andrew Weil that the less protein we eat, the less protein there is for our immune systems to attack.[10]

I believe the diet I have created for myself has helped me recover from lupus. I eat plant protein provided by grains, green vegetables, and some legumes. I also eat between 10 and 20 percent animal protein, excluding red meat. The source of my animal protein is cold-water, ocean-going fish, like salmon and halibut, and organically grown chicken. I minimize animal protein in my daily meals by cutting fish fillets and skinned chicken pieces into three-ounce servings. Nutritionists tell us that four, three-ounce servings of animal protein a week is enough to keep us healthy. We eat vegetarian meals the other three days per week.

Avoiding Foods That Make Us Worse

People with lupus often have a specific allergy to an amino acid called L-canavanine, which is found in all legumes. For years I thought I was imagining not being able to eat green peas or chickpeas without feeling nauseous. Then I learned about L-canavanine and suspected that I had the sensitivity. Avoiding those two legumes has helped me feel better.

I also thought that I was allergic to alfalfa sprouts, but now I understand they make me nauseous and dizzy because they contain L-canavanine as well. Researchers now know that lupus patients should avoid alfalfa sprouts strictly, because they actually can cause lupus flare-ups in particularly sensitive people. Avoidance is harder than one might imagine, however, since alfalfa is an ingredient in many food products and some natural vitamin supplements.[11] Be sure to read food and vitamin labels carefully. Even then you may not catch all the sources of alfalfa. Years ago I was eating organically grown beef, thinking it would help me feel better, but I was feeling progressively worse. Querying the farmer who had raised the beef, I learned that he had fed alfalfa to those cattle. When I stopped eating the meat that contained alfalfa, I felt better.

Other foods lupus patients may need to avoid include peanuts, soybeans, and lentils. In addition, The National Institute of Arthritic, Musculoskeletal, and Skin Diseases stated in 1996 that "recent evidence suggests that corn, spinach, and carrots may aggravate the symptoms of lupus."[12] There are various theories about why these particular vegetables can make us worse, but no one knows the answer for certain. The best way to test your ability to tolerate them is to eat each vegetable, one at a time, away from other food. Wait a few hours, and if you still feel well, it is a good sign that you're not sensitive to that particular food.

I also suspect that we lupus patients may be sensitive to sulfur-containing vegetables. I have difficulty eating cabbage, brussels sprouts, broccoli, kale, and cauliflower, all of which are cruciferous vegetables containing high levels of organic sulfur compounds. I can eat small quantities of them in raw form, but when they're cooked they nauseate me. Cooking changes the chemical composition of these foods. We know that many of us with lupus are sensitive to sulfa drugs, so it seems reasonable to suspect that sulfa sensitivity carries over into sulfur-containing foods. If you feel worse when you eat cruciferous vegetables, avoiding them may be wise.

If you have lupus and you drink coffee, tea, or cola, it's imperative that you stop. These are all caffeinated beverages, and caffeine is an extremely toxic substance for the body to metabolize. What's more, coffee, even the decaffeinated variety, is one of the most disruptive substances in relation to the smooth flow of liver chi. Many of us feel a tightness in our shoulder and neck muscles after ingesting this powerful stimulant. TCM teaches that it can be extremely difficult for people who drink coffee, either regular or decaf, to resolve liver imbalances.[13]

Because caffeine is a stimulant, it can add to your stress by increasing your heart rate. We know that stress is a primary cause of lupus flare-ups. Caffeine also can lead to stomach problems. Withdrawing from caffeine slowly over a week can cushion you from the severe headaches and irritability that can result from caffeine withdrawal. Here is a suggestion that may help you withdraw from coffee. Drink only one cup per day for three days. Drink one-half cup decaffeinated coffee mixed with a half cup caffeinated coffee for the next two days. On the sixth and seventh days, drink one-quarter caffeinated and three-quarters decaffeinated coffee mixed. By the second week you should feel fine.[14] Even though some health professionals think drinking decaf coffee is harmless, I strongly disagree. Not only should lupus patients stop drinking all caffeinated beverages, but we should stop drinking coffee altogether.

Most tea is caffeinated, as are soft drinks like Coca-Cola, Tab, Royal Crown (RC) Cola, Dr. Pepper, Mountain Dew, and Pepsi, though some manufacturers finally are offering caffeine-free varieties. None of these drinks are good for us, not only because of their caffeine but also because of their high sugar content. Read labels very carefully. Better than drinking any of them is drinking herbal teas and vegetable broths instead. At our house, we created a new drink. We mix two or three tablespoons frozen fruit juice concentrate in a glass of sparkling water and call it a "tropical sunset." Our guests delight in these natural home-mixed sodas.

Drinking even small amounts of alcohol is not a good idea for lupus patients. Even though the popular press has reported alcohol's possible beneficial effects against heart disease, the fact is that alcohol ingestion is potentially dangerous. It is a poison and even small amounts, consumed regularly, can cause damage to the body, particularly the liver. Repeated consumption of alcohol inhibits the liver's production of digestive enzymes, which in turn impairs the body's ability to absorb protein, fat, and the fat-soluble vitamins A, D, E, and K, as well as B-complex vitamins, especially thiamine and folic acid.[15]

Well-documented evidence indicates that alcohol may increase serum estradiol, a female hormone suspected of causing cancer, by 300 percent in postmenopausal women who were taking hormone replacement therapy. Alcohol also increases the incidence of breast cancer, osteoporosis, depression, pancreatitis, liver cirrhosis, gastritis, degenerative nervous system conditions, fetus damage (fetal alcohol syndrome), substance abuse, and cancers of the mouth, pharynx, larynx, esophagus, and liver.[16] In addition, severe behavior problems may result from drinking alcohol. Avoiding alcohol would seem to be the best practice for anyone trying to recover from a chronic illness such as lupus.

In my opinion, the worst food we eat is refined sugar. There are many kinds of sugars, including the most common one—table sugar, or sucrose. Other sugars are raw sugar, dextrose (corn sugar), fructose, honey, brown sugar, maple syrup, molasses, corn syrups, milk sugar (or lactose), and sorbitol. Each of us seems to handle and react differently to these sugars. The primary problem with sugar is that it is potentially highly allergy-inducing and addictive. It plays a major role in the pathogenesis of diabetes and hypoglycemia and may also produce anxiety, high cholesterol and triglycerides, ulcers, depression, hyperactivity, hypertension, and mental and nervous system disorders.

Refined sugars lack all the essential nutrients necessary for their metabolization. This means that our bodies have to cannibalize our own nutrients to digest sugars. This process particularly stresses our livers. Even worse, sugar inhibits our immune response by impairing the activity of our "scavenger" white blood cells that fight disease. Americans today consume more than 125 pounds of processed sugar per year. Only 150 years ago, an ordinary person ate ten pounds of sugar or less. It seems clear to me that those of us with lupus should avoid sugar, under its many aliases, altogether. It is much too detrimental to our health to continue eating it. Is it realistic to think we can avoid sugar? The answer is yes, if you're willing to switch to mild sweeteners that do not raise your blood glucose levels. Even mild sweeteners (fruit juice concentrate or brown rice syrup) should be used in moderation, however.

Removing sugar from our diets can be challenging, because it is so addictive and prevalent in many canned, packaged, and processed foods. At the time my illness struck, I craved ice cream and chocolate bars. But after I learned about the dangers of sugar, I stopped eating it. Then I plummeted cold turkey into the "sugar blues," which lasted about ten days. Now I feel much better not eating sugar. When I do eat it occasionally, I am sometimes dizzy and weak for a few hours. Eliminating sugar from your diet will take determination and persistence. You may feel worse for a while, but take heart. If you eat lots of vegetables, grains, and some protein during the withdrawal, you will begin to feel significantly better than you felt when you still ate sugar.

There are four nonsugar products we use in our home that safeguard us from sugar binges. One of these sweeteners is called stevia. This plant, which is part of the chrysanthemum family, grows primarily in South America and China. It serves in much of the world as a food and beverage sweetener. A benefit of stevia is that it seems to balance the blood glucose. Because it is not a sugar, it does not raise insulin levels in the way sugar does. It also may have anti-inflammatory capabilities that can benefit lupus patients. Stevia is so strong in its liquid form that you must use it only by the drop. A delicious breakfast recipe using stevia calls for one diced apple, one and a half teaspoons chopped walnuts, one-half cup 1 percent cottage cheese, and three drops stevia. Mix together and enjoy.

In dry form, stevia comes in white or green powder. Though white stevia is significantly more expensive than green stevia, it is much tastier. Mix the powder at a proportion of one teaspoon stevia to six teaspoons water. Then add it to your herbal tea by the drop. Use one teaspoon of stevia for one cup of white sugar in recipes. The white stevia is best for most baked goods, but you can use the green stevia in muffins and darker cakes. A drawback of stevia is that it does not tenderize baked goods as refined sugar does. It is also expensive by the pound, but remember that a small amount of this herb goes a long way. The benefits of stevia far outweigh its limitations. Be willing to experiment with it. It is available in food co-ops and health food stores.

Another possible sugar substitute is fructose. This simple sugar that comes from corn does not raise blood glucose levels as refined cane sugar does. It has only a low impact on blood glucose, such as soybeans have.[17]

You can bake with fructose by simply substituting it for refined sugar in your recipes. Do not use fructose if you are allergic to corn. It is available in powdered form at your local food co-op.

If used in moderation, brown rice syrup will not raise your blood glucose levels as sucrose does. It has a mild flavor. To replace one cup of refined sugar in a recipe, use three-fourths cup brown rice syrup. You may have to increase the amount of dry ingredients a bit. This simple brownie recipe incorporating brown rice syrup is delicious.

Sift together:

   2 cups flour
   $1/_2$ cup cocoa powder
   $1^1/_4$ teaspoons baking soda
   $1/_2$ teaspoon salt

Beat together, in order:
   2 eggs
   $1/_4$ cup canola oil
   1 cup plus 2 tablespoons brown rice syrup
   $1/_2$ cup warm water
   2 tablespoons real vanilla

Mix wet and dry ingredients together thoroughly. Pour the mixture into an oiled pan, 8 x 8 x $1/_2$ inch. Bake in a 350-degree oven for forty to fifty minutes. These brownies are done when a knife pressed in the middle of the pan comes out clean. Be careful not to overbake or they will be too dry.

You can also replace cane sugar with fruit juice concentrate. Be cautioned that it may change the flavor of baked goods a bit. Use the juice concentrate frozen as it comes out of the container. If your recipe calls for one cup sugar, replace it with one-half cup frozen juice concentrate. As with brown rice syrup, you may have to increase the amount of dry ingredients.

Nutritionists tell us to eat a lot of fruit, but at least one nutritionist I've worked with says Americans eat too much fruit. In his opinion, all this fruit is detrimental to us, because it raises our blood glucose levels. When I reduced my fruit intake by cutting back to one piece of raw fruit a day, I didn't notice that I felt better, and I craved fruit because I enjoy it so much. In addition, not all fruit is alike. Some, like dates, raisins, figs, and other dried fruits, have higher glycemic levels. I don't know how much fruit we can eat safely, but, in general, eating fewer sweeteners, whether natural or refined, is a healthy thing to do.

EATING GOOD FOOD FOR BETTER HEALTH

For all the reasons I have stated, I believe that it's very important for lupus patients to eat an alkaline diet. Vegetable broth, vegetable juice, and fruit juice are all high-alkaline foods and, as such, offer great restorative help for lupus patients. What foods other than soups and juices can we eat to maintain high alkalinity? Nutritious foods high in alkalinity include figs, soybeans, lima beans, apricots, spinach, turnips, beets, raisins, almonds, carrots, dates, celery, and cucumber. Be aware that turnips, beets, raisins, dates, and carrots are foods with high glycemic indexes as well. Neutral acid foods are milk, butter, vegetable oils, and white sugar. To maintain our body's alkalinity, we need to eat fewer high-acid foods, including oysters, veal, most fish, liver, chicken, most red meats, eggs, most grains, rice, and most nuts, except almonds and Brazil nuts.

If we decide to eat animal protein and want to eat fish, it's best to eat cold-water, ocean-going fish, such as salmon, red snapper, and halibut. The danger of eating fish that's higher on the food chain, such as shark, swordfish, and tuna is that these fish may contain more concentrated levels of environmental pollutants than smaller fish. This approach will not safeguard us completely, however; there is now evidence that all our fish populations are contaminated with varying levels of pollutants.

Another creative way to supplement a healthy diet is to eat wild greens that grow in North America, such as dandelion greens, lamb's-quarter, purslane, chickweed, watercress, and nettles, which is an important immune enhancer. These greens grow all around us in the spring and summer, often on our own properties. Going "greens gathering" with friends can be a pleasant way to spend an afternoon.

Here is a recipe for "wild greens powder" that you can make in the spring and use on your food as a tonic during the long winter months, to help enhance your resistance to infections. Locate unsprayed sources of the following wild plants, making certain you can identify them correctly: yellow dock *(Rumex crispus)*, mallow (*Malva* species), dandelion *(Taraxacum)*, chicory *(Chickorium officinale)*, plantain (*Plantago* species), and nettles (*Urtica* species). Pick only undamaged, green, healthy leaves of several species of these or others that are available in your area. Dry the leaves in a commercial dryer or by hanging them in a dry place where air can circulate around them for a few weeks. Then, using a mortar and pestle, grind them to a powder and store in an amber glass jar. Sprinkle on your food.

Another good food we need in our diets is fat. Too much saturated fat can be difficult for the liver to break down, but some fat is necessary for our bodies to function efficiently. Although advice on the best fats to eat has differed widely lately, I've learned that the best sources of beneficial fat are olive oil, flaxseed oil, and raw nuts and seeds. Olive oil is resistant to oxidation and contains a good balance of saturated, monounsaturated, and unsaturated fatty acids. Flax oil, also called linseed oil, is rich in essential fatty, linoleic, and linolenic acids. Raw nuts and seeds are an excellent source of high-quality essential fatty acids and have low amounts of saturated fat. See chapter 7 for specifics on beneficial fats and oils.

Drinking Safe Water

The quality of the water we drink is critically important. In my attempt to recover my health by minimizing the stress on my body, I wondered whether I was drinking enough water. I also wondered about the quality of that water. Although I drank large volumes of water in Africa to guard against dehydration, I realized that I may have stopped drinking enough water after I left the oppressive heat of East Africa. Wondering whether I might be somewhat dehydrated, I decided to remedy that by drinking more water.

Drinking sufficient water is vital, because water allows the body to function effectively. It is of great importance to lupus patients, in particular, because it cleanses the blood by removing wastes through the kidneys. Water also helps regulate body temperature through perspiration. Without enough water, our bodies cannot digest or metabolize food. Too little water also can affect the nervous system's ability to send nerve impulses to the brain and muscles. Inadequate water can lessen blood volume, thereby limiting the oxygen and nutrients provided to all our muscles and organs.[18]

As a chronically ill person, I have tried to drink a minimum of ten glasses of water a day since shortly after I became ill. Among my family and friends I have become known as the "serious water drinker." They often hand me glasses, cups, or pitchers of water without my even asking. Some of them have told me that my dedication to drinking water has raised their consciousness about drinking enough water, too.

During my illness, I had sensitivities to some metals and was so concerned about picking up bacteria from water that I chose to drink distilled water for two years, hoping to avoid those contaminants. I now think that was a mistake, because distillation removes the minerals from water. I began drinking nondistilled, filtered water again to obtain the trace minerals I need. If you can't manage to drink ten glasses of water a day, you can replace a portion of your daily water intake with herbal tea, natural fruit juices, and some soups. It's best not to substitute such drinks as soda, processed fruit juices, coffee, or tea for your daily water ration, however, because they contain many chemicals that are difficult for your body to metabolize.

Water safety is an important issue for all of us today. The health of our drinking water varies greatly in this country. The water in industrialized areas, for example, can be unsafe to drink. In a city just forty miles away from us the soil and water have been contaminated for years by arsenic spewing from an aluminum smelter. Federal Environmental Protection Agency studies have verified that the cancer rate in that community is abnormally high. In my community, however, in addition to treated water that is chlorinated, we have artesian well water available that is sweet, safe, and free. A local nonprofit group known as Friends of Artesians raises money to maintain the well and monitor its water quality. The group is even planning to develop a small city park around the well. People line up at the spigot, chatting and laughing as they await their turns to fill their bottles with the deep, delicious, uncontaminated water.

Some of us living in rural areas still have our own wells that supply pure water that we do not have to treat with chlorine. Chlorine can be a problem for many of us who are chemically sensitive. Two of the worst water contaminants are lead and radon. Even a high iron content in water can pose potential health problems. Water may contain bacterial contaminants as well. Beware of coliform bacteria, which comes from human and animal waste and can seep into the water table where septic systems leak or animal herds graze. If you are ill, it is a good idea to have your water tested wherever you live. Call your county or state health department for referrals to labs that test water. At best, you will find that your water is safe to drink. If it is not safe, you should consider treating your water and using a water filter. Talk to your local health officer and read *Consumer Reports* to find the best filter. If you do nothing else, purchasing an inexpensive carafe-style water filter can benefit you by providing at least 50 percent safer, tastier water.

On my safari through alternative nutritional practices, I learned many new approaches to eating for health. Today my husband and I continue to eat carefully. Avoiding fat and sugar as much as possible, we eat a lot of broth and large quantities of raw and steamed vegetables along with pasta, bulgur, brown rice, cold-water fish, and organically grown chicken once a week. We eat only small portions of fresh fruit. We rarely eat packaged, processed, frozen, or fast foods, other than the occasional pizza. I still crave sugar, chocolate, butter, and ice cream from time to time, but I eat them only rarely. My doctors sometimes comment on my excellent blood pressure and low cholesterol and triglyceride levels. Their positive reinforcement encourages me to move through my food cravings and continue to eat wisely. My journey into learning about how foods affect us has taught me that, as lupus patients, we can improve our health by eating more alkaline, plant-based diets.

5

Helpful Nutritional Supplements

The best treatment is the least—the least invasive, least drastic, least expensive—that activates spontaneous healing.

Andrew Weil, M.D.

Ten years ago, in the deep days of my illness, I remember walking unsteadily around our organic gardens arm in arm with a friend, wondering aloud, "How can I recover my strength and resilience? Is there anything safe and natural that will help me?" "Why don't you try nutritional supplements?" he answered. When I asked two conventional physicians about nutritional supplements for lupus, neither of them offered any suggestions. After my second attempt, it occurred to me that these doctors probably didn't know anything about the application of natural supplements to chronic illness.

Many of us are aware that allopathic physicians know little about nutritional supplements. Indeed, most of them generally advise patients that nutritional supplements will not relieve their symptoms. Their professional organization, the American Medical Association (AMA), officially states that there is no evidence that supplements improve our health and that they may even harm us. An example of this position appears in a recent article on diet and cancer published by the Center for Science in the Public Interest. The medical doctor who was interviewed stated, "Dietary supplements are probably unnecessary, and possibly unhelpful, for reducing cancer risk." "Unhelpful" is defined in a footnote as meaning "harmful."[1] Some of us wonder whether the AMA takes this position on supplements because it works so closely with the American pharmaceutical industry.

Whether all American medical doctors believe that nutritional supplements are ineffective is another issue. I have been a guest in one allopathic physician's home, where I saw bottles of vitamin supplements crowding a kitchen cupboard, yet this man does not recommend nutritional supplements to his patients. Two other medical doctors have told me that they and their families take vitamins and minerals each day, but they don't recommend natural medicines to their patients because of the AMA's official position on nutritional supplements.

There are other professional views, however, that focus on the great potential of natural supplements to help us. Most naturopaths we know emphasize healthy diets, supplements, and herbs as an integral part of their families' lives. Dining in the home of a TCM practitioner recently, we learned about the healing herbal broths that provide many nutrients to her family. Visiting with all of these families has reinforced my certainty that it is important to stay open and curious about healing options.

My own twelve-year safari through natural healing contradicts the American allopathic medical position on nutritional supplements. On my journey toward wellness, I have found nine nutritional supplements that have helped diminish my lupus symptoms. These are biochemic tissue salts, glandular extracts, magnesium, vitamin A, vitamin C, Coenzyme Q-10, D,L-phenylalanine (DLPA), L-tyrosine, and dehydroepiandrosterone (DHEA). Speaking from my own experience, I know these supplements hold great promise for positively affecting body chemistry to encourage healing of lupus.

BIOCHEMIC TISSUE SALTS

One of the most important concepts in wellness is that healthy cells do not become diseased. Once I understood this, I began searching for a low-cost, safe, easy-to-use system of natural medication that could help reestablish my cellular health and thereby lessen my lupus symptoms. When I found biochemic tissue salts, I knew they fit my needs perfectly. These tissue salts are the twelve biochemical components that cells need to stay healthy. I have had good results using homeopathic tissue salts to minimize muscle and joint pain, anxiety, and nervousness associated with my lupus. These tiny pills also seemed to diminish my sleeplessness, depression, and cold hands and feet.

When I discovered these little salts, I wanted to learn more about their origins. In 1873 a German doctor of medicine, William H. Schuessler, began to publish a series of articles on the subject of body tissue salts. He studied and defined the function of each of the twelve basic tissue salts and carefully detailed the disorders he thought would arise if any of these salts was deficient. Through my reading, I learned that biochemic salts are used in ways that are both similar to and different from the ways that homeopathic medicines are used. Homeopaths use almost any active substance—even poisons—in minute concentrations. Biochemical therapists, on the other hand, use only those inorganic salts that occur naturally in the body. However, like homeopaths, biochemical therapists use these substances in very dilute concentrations.

You may be wondering, as I did, just how such minute quantities of tissue salts could have the capacity to heal us? Although there is no easy explanation, researchers are getting closer to an answer. Knowledge from the field of quantum mechanics, which works on the assumption that energy, rather than mass, is at the heart of everything, in combination with research in biochemistry may hold the answer. The research suggests that even if few of the original molecules of a substance are left, the fluid in which the molecules were originally dissolved might still carry information, in the form of energy, about the original substance. So the tissue salt remedy exists at a low concentration but a high intrinsic energy state.

66

Scientists think this high intrinsic energy stimulates various bioenergetic systems in the body.

Quantum mechanics also suggests that these imprinted energy patterns have self-replicating qualities. It's possible, therefore, that biochemic tissue salts and homeopathic remedies work so well because they actually "reproduce" in the bioenergetic systems of the body, thereby helping our bodies fight disease.[2] This research has helped me understand that biochemic tissue salts seem to supercharge existing biochemical pathways in our bodies that involve the inorganic salts.

You can use tissue salts in two ways. They are particularly useful for short-lived, self-limiting conditions, sometimes producing results in acute illness, such as the flu, in only a few hours. The salts also can be helpful in chronic conditions, but then it may take weeks or even months of treatment to correct the mineral deficiency that is contributing to the chronic illness.

Tissue salts sounded like such a good idea that I knew I would be using them over the long term to treat my serious and deep-seated chronic illness. I had a number of symptoms, including poor circulation, depression, nervousness, anxiety, and sleeplessness, all of which, I learned through my research, might be treatable with *Kalium phosphoricum,* or Kali. phos., (from the mineral potassium phosphate). I took the remedy for three months before I noticed my nervousness and anxiety beginning to slowly dissipate. I also felt the circulation returning to my hands and feet, which had been cold for many years, and my muscle and joint pain began to subside.

Since I believe that lupus originates on a cellular level, it seems to me that tissue salts, with their ability to rebalance cellular health, may benefit SLE patients. You'll be pleased to know that, in the form of tiny white pills, biochemic tissue salts are inexpensive and completely safe. One cautionary note is that because the tissue salts are diluted with milk sugar, people with lactose intolerance may have difficulty with tissue salt therapy. Other than that, there are no known side effects.

To determine the appropriate tissue salt for you, you'll need to be aware of specific symptoms you want to treat. Then, using a reference text on tissue salts, determine which salt will treat your symptom or set of symptoms.[3]

You may need to use more than one salt. Take the number of tablets rec-ommended on the label of the bottle, letting them dissolve under your tongue. For my pain, I used a combination of *Magnesia phosphorica* (Mag. phos.), Kali. phos., and Ferrum phosphoricum (Ferrum phos.), each at 6× concentration. Take four tablets of each tissue salt three times a day for a minimum of three months to begin to experience benefit from the salts. Biochemic tissue salts are available at many health food stores and bulk herb outlets. If your local stores do not carry tissue salts, ask them to spe-cial order the salts for you.

GLANDULAR EXTRACTS

The stress lupus puts on our bodies undoubtedly depletes our reservoirs of nutrients. When we are ill, the glandular system needs superior nourishment, because all our bodily processes are dependent on properly functioning glands to secrete the necessary levels of hormones into the bloodstream. Vitamins and minerals, as well as glandular extracts, can help support the glandular system, which in turn can strengthen us.

Probably the most important endocrine glands for lupus patients are the thymus and the spleen.[4] The thymus is the overseer of the immune system, but in many adults it is relatively inactive or completely atrophied. Although orthodox medicine thinks that this shrinking of the thymus is normal, the field of naturopathy emphasizes that we need strong thymus glands all of our lives. Holistic nutritionists believe that thymus atrophy may stem from improper diet. The thymus needs vitamins A, B_6, and C and the minerals zinc, iron, and selenium, as well as the essential fatty acids, to perform its tasks well. The typical American diet is deficient in many of these nutrients. A healthy thymus gland is particularly important for those of us with lupus. T lymphocytes, the antibodies that fight infection, are formed in the thymus gland. T-lymphocyte levels often are suppressed in lupus patients, which may be part of the reason we are susceptible to infections.

Another gland that is a critical component of the immune system is the spleen. It's important to understand the basic tasks of the spleen in order to comprehend its great importance to lupus patients. This gland is composed of lymphoid tissue and produces white blood cells, which clean up the blood. On one level, lupus is a blood disease, and so it would follow that a strong spleen may help us recover from lupus. The spleen sends the debris from the blood into the lymphatic system, where the lymph nodes kill the bacteria that have been disabled by the white cells. This lymph waste then is excreted through the skin in the form of perspiration and through urine and feces. The spleen functions in conjunction with the liver. It needs the essential fatty acids, B vitamins, and vitamin C as well as selenium, zinc, and iron to be strong enough on a cellular level to perform its many tasks.

Another way to strengthen the glands, in addition to taking vitamins and minerals, is by taking glandular extracts—concentrated forms of beef and sheep glands. Naturopaths may use glandular extracts as one of many possible treatments for patients with chronic illness. When my naturopath suggested them to me, I wanted to learn about them before I made a decision to take them. My reading revealed that clinicians were perplexed for decades about how glandular extracts work. Then, in the 1930s, a biochemical researcher named Dr. Royal Lee developed an amazing theory. He suggested that human organs malfunction because the immune system attacks them in a subtle way, thereby causing chronic health problems. Dr. Lee's pioneering research showed that glandular extracts neutralize these attacks by the immune system, allowing the organs to heal and rebalance.

More recent research has verified Dr. Lee's work. Glandular extracts seem to work on an energy level, moving through the biochemical pathways in the same way biochemic tissue salts do.[5] The implications of this research are extremely important for autoimmune disease. Could it be that many people who are chronically ill are experiencing an autoimmune illness? Could it also be that this autoimmune response is occurring at such a subtle level that current laboratory tests do not pick it up? And could it be that these patients would be helped by glandular extracts, if they took them early enough to prevent their illnesses from becoming full-blown? This line of questioning suggests that early on in our disease, when our conditions were much less severe, those of us with autoimmune illnesses might have been treatable with glandular extracts had laboratory tests been able to verify this subtle autoimmune attack syndrome.

At the suggestion of two naturopaths, I took thymus glandular extract for about one year during the worst phase of my illness, and I believe that it helped me gain enough physical strength to start walking fifteen minutes a day. I did not take spleen extract during those years, because the naturopaths did not suggest it. But now, with my increased understanding of how glandular extracts work, I think that a combination of spleen and thymus extracts has the potential to help lupus patients.

Although glandular extracts generally are considered safe, one naturopath with whom I have worked is concerned about their raw state. She believes that there could be pathogens in the raw granular form of the gland. Other practitioners I've talked with say freeze-drying kills any pathogens. You will need to make your own decision about whether to take them. If you decide to use these extracts, be sure to consult a naturopath or holistic physician who is skilled in using them. And be careful to purchase only extracts that have come from young, free-range, organically grown animals that have not been fed antibiotics or hormones. At present, there is a source of glandular extracts imported from New Zealand that meet these screening criteria.

Magnesium

Magnesium is critically important for those of us with lupus for a number of reasons. Continuing with our theme that cellular health is the key to healing, it is imperative that our cells have adequate magnesium to perform their functions efficiently. Magnesium is needed as a cofactor of essential fatty acid metabolism. Insufficient magnesium in the body can cause arthritis pain, elevated cholesterol levels, premenstrual syndrome, high blood pressure, lowered body metabolism and temperature, asthma, obesity, and hyperactivity. It also can provoke muscle weakness, irritability, even convulsions.

I have a theory that many of us with autoimmune disease may have impaired enzyme systems for making magnesium, calcium, and potassium available to our cells. The resulting deficiencies of these minerals weaken us, making us more vulnerable to illness. During the worst years of my lupus, I was nervous, exhausted, and weak. It was some years later that I started to take 600 mg a day of magnesium citrate and realized, within a few weeks, that it was beginning to help me. I became calmer and more able to focus on people and activities around me. I slowly regained my ability to understand what I was reading, and I could follow conversations more easily. Very gradually I also began to feel physically stronger, able at that point to walk more than fifteen minutes at a time, and to hoe and weed my gardens for fifteen to thirty minutes twice a week. My leg muscles began to stop aching and cramping, and I slowly grew to feel less fatigued, though I still needed many hours of rest each day.

Six years of taking magnesium has helped me so much that I plan to take the supplement for the rest of my life. It is possible to get enough magnesium in food if we eat lots of green, leafy vegetables, nuts, peas, and beans. Deficiencies can develop if our diets are too high in saturated fats, or if we eat too much processed food or too many dairy products, which creates an excess of calcium in our systems. We also may need extra-large doses of magnesium if our bodies aren't able to metabolize it efficiently.

If you take no other supplement, start taking magnesium, because it has a strong potential for helping you feel better over the long term. This supplement should be taken in a ratio of two parts magnesium to three parts calcium.[6] The recommended daily dosage of magnesium is 350 mg minimum and twice that amount or more for therapeutic purposes. These quantities are safe unless you have kidney symptoms associated with lupus. Magnesium oxide is poorly absorbed. Some of the most easily assimilated forms of magnesium are fumate, malate, citrate, and glycinate—these types are bound to amino acids for better absorption. If you have kidney failure or are suffering from Addison disease or myasthenia gravis, you should not take supplemental magnesium.[7]

Vitamin A

Many of us learned as teenagers that we need vitamin A, also called retinoic acid, for healthy skin. In the past two decades, published research has shown the beneficial effects of vitamin A on the epidermis and epidermal linings of the body. Vitamin A can be a great help to those of us with lupus, because it can safeguard the thymus gland and even promote its growth. A strong thymus supports a strong immune response, which makes vitamin A a potent virus fighter. This vitamin is synthesized from carotenes, which are orange plant pigments, and can protect us against epithelial cancers of the skin, gastrointestinal tract, and lungs. Many people today take beta-carotene rather than vitamin A, but my experience has been with the vitamin itself, supplemented with natural beta-carotene in my diet. Good food sources of carotenes include colored root vegetables, such as carrots, sweet potatoes and yams, broccoli, winter squash and all green, leafy vegetables.[8]

On my journey through the research on vitamin A, I found one study that has important significance for lupus patients. Vitamin A appears to possess immunomodulatory activity, meaning that it can balance the immune response. In a study done on lupus patients in Hungary in 1987, researchers verified that vitamin A therapy can partially restore depressed cellular immune reactivity in patients with SLE. Patients were given 100,000 IU of vitamin A daily for two weeks. This dose enhanced their natural killer cell activity as well as their levels of ADCC, or antibody-dependent cell-mediated cytotoxicity. Both of these beneficial immune responses are suppressed in lupus patients, which is why they tend to have many viral and bacterial infections. Researchers in this study stated that the effect of vitamin A therapy on immune reactivity, susceptibility to viral infections, and survival in patients with SLE requires further study.[9] I have supplemented my diet with 25,000 IU daily of vitamin A for eight years. Based on the Hungarian research alone, I believe this inexpensive vitamin may have the potential to help anyone with lupus. Do not exceed 25,000 IU without checking with a naturopath or holistic physician, because vitamin A can be toxic at high levels.

VITAMIN C

Vitamin C is extremely important for those of us with lupus. When our family veterinarian mentioned that dogs produce their own vitamin C and consequently don't need the supplement in their diets, I wondered about human beings' need for vitamin C. Could it be that our species also may have produced its own vitamin C but over the millennia lost that ability? The physicist and Nobel laureate Dr. Linus Pauling wrote extensively about our need for supplemental vitamin C to strengthen our immune response and protect us from disease.

Vitamin C is an antioxidant that protects our cells from free-radical damage, thus slowing the aging process. Free radicals are oxidized reactive atoms that are highly destructive to our tissues. Very important for lupus patients, vitamin C has anti-inflammatory action.[10] It also lowers blood histamine levels, which cause allergic reactions, and, for this reason, is a good treatment for allergies. Moreover, it can help lower cholesterol, triglyceride, and total fat levels, while elevating the level of high-density lipoproteins, which sweep the body clean of excess cholesterol. Vitamin C can stimulate secretion of thymus hormones and, very important for lupus patients, restore the integrity of connective tissue.

I took 10 g of vitamin C a day for four years; now I take 6 g a day as a maintenance dose. I think that it protects me during the winter cold and flu season. It's important to know that the high concentration of vitamin C in white blood cells is rapidly depleted when we have an infection; a vitamin C deficiency may ensue if ascorbic acid is not replenished regularly. When we're sick, we need to take supplemental vitamin C to replenish our stores. If the acid in vitamin C preparations irritates your stomach, try taking the sodium ascorbate form of vitamin C, which is buffered. Although it is rare to be allergic to vitamin C, start with low doses to make certain you can tolerate it.

Lendon Smith, M.D., author of *Feed Yourself Right*, states that lupus patients should take 10 g (10,000 mg) of vitamin C per day to help the adrenal glands produce natural cortisol, which can strengthen us and reduce our fatigue levels.[11] Vitamin C is easily lost when food is cooked or processed, so it is important to eat raw fruits and leafy, green vegetables each day to obtain adequate natural vitamin C.

COENZYME Q-10

Also known as ubiqunone and CoQ-10, this enzyme is essential for the health of all our tissues and organs. When we are young and healthy, our bodies generally produce enough CoQ-10 to protect us, but as we age we often generate less of this enzyme than we need. CoQ-10 performs a critical function in manufacturing adenosine triphosphate, the basic energy molecule of the cell. It carries oxygen into the mitochondria, or "heart," of each cell, thereby increasing cellular energy. CoQ-10 is an antioxidant that protects cells against free radicals, which cause our cells to age. The heart and liver need high concentrations of CoQ-10. Because it is pivotal to cellular metabolism, a deficiency of CoQ-10 may provoke the development of many different conditions, such as cardiovascular disease and age-related deterioration of the immune system. We may be able to protect ourselves from some of the effects of aging by taking CoQ-10.

The case is very strong for taking CoQ-10 when we are ill with lupus. Tissue-injury diseases such as lupus—on one level a connective tissue disorder—may respond to CoQ-10 treatment, because this enzyme is an antioxidant that can stop oxygen radicals from damaging the tissue.[12] When we have autoimmune conditions, our weakened bodies sometimes have more difficulty fighting off pathogens. What may be a simple cold or mild case of flu for a person with a healthy immune system can result in pneumonia or even death for some of us who are already ill when the pathogen attacks. CoQ-10 stimulates the macrophages to fight off invaders; therefore, CoQ-10 has antibacterial and antitumor effects.

Periodontal disease, a weak heart, and severe fatigue were symptoms of my lupus. Ten years ago I was unable to find a local health practitioner who knew anything about this enzyme, but my journey through the European research suggested that CoQ-10 might offer me some relief. The alternative physician I found and consulted with by phone in another part of the state suggested that I take up to 60 mg of CoQ-10 a day. I was so ill when I started taking it that I raised the dose to 260 mg a day before I felt any improvement. At that dose, CoQ-10 finally began to help me feel better. Over many months of supplementation with this enzyme, my gums stopped swelling and bleeding, my heart palpitations became less pronounced, and my energy level improved.

CoQ-10 is expensive, because it is imported from Japan. If you would like to replenish this enzyme in your body but are unable to purchase it in supplement form, you may be able to increase your CoQ-10 levels dietarily. Try eating more rice bran, wheat germ, soybeans, almonds, pistachios, hazelnuts, broccoli, sweet potatoes, carrots, cauliflower, beef, and sardines. These are all excellent sources of CoQ-10. There are no known side effects of CoQ-10, and there is no toxicity if you take it as a supplement. You can feel safe taking this enzyme for the rest of your life if you think that it helps you. In rare cases, a person is allergic to it, so raise your dose gradually. A maintenance dosage is 10 to 30 mg per day. The therapeutic dosage for people with lupus would be up to and above 100 mg per day.

DLPA AND L-TYROSINE

These two amino acids have a specific potential for helping those of us with autoimmune conditions. Although I could find no studies concerning DLPA and lupus, I believe that my experience with it shows that it can help lupus patients, depending on specific symptoms. A natural amino acid, DLPA, also known as D,L-phenylalanine, can be an effective pain reliever for the chronic pain of osteoarthritis, rheumatoid arthritis, lower back pain, and migraine headaches. It appears to work by inhibiting the breakdown of endorphins, which are mild mood elevators and potent pain relievers, thereby enhancing the effect of endorphins in the body's own pain-relieving system.[13]

Some naturopaths use DLPA in clinical practice for treating both pain and depression. I had a great deal of pain and depression until I found DLPA, and my naturopath agreed that I should try it. Within two weeks, I began experiencing less pain and a moderately elevated mood. One allopathic physician I discovered uses DLPA, too. Patricia Slagle, M.D., a psychiatrist, has treated many cases of depression successfully with a combination of L-tyrosine and DLPA. In addition to these two amino acids, she also prescribes vitamin B complex, vitamin C, and a daily multivitamin/mineral capsule to treat depression.

From my own experience, I would suggest that these amino acids can offer an alternative for treating the pain and depression that often accompany lupus. Using them could allow you to avoid the expensive and potentially toxic pharmaceuticals that are now available for treating depression. You can start with 500 mg to 1,000 mg of L-tyrosine when you get up in the morning and again in the midafternoon. Do not take this amino acid with any protein food, because you will absorb less of it if you do. Take it with water, juice, or fruit and wait at least thirty minutes before you eat protein. Take 500 to 600 mg at bedtime with a complex carbohydrate, such as whole grain bread, which will allow it to be better absorbed. Do not eat sugar, fruit, or fruit juices at night, because they can cause sleep disturbances. If your pain level and depression don't improve in two weeks, gradually raise the dosage of L-tyrosine, but do not exceed 3,500 mg per day. When your depression is alleviated and your pain is lessened, stay at that dosage.

Deficiencies of any of the B vitamins can lead to depression, so supplementing with vitamin B complex is important. Try to buy B complex in powder or capsules since it is digested more easily. Use the coated form of B_6, so that it is not destroyed by stomach acid. If the pyridoxal 5-phosphate form of B_6 doesn't appear in your B_6 formula, you'll need to purchase it separately and take 20 to 120 mg twice daily. Take a multivitamin and mineral capsule in the morning and evening.[14]

According to Dr. Slagle, this program should treat depression successfully. If it doesn't work, or if you have pain along with depression at the outset, you'll need to add DLPA to the protocol. Use 1,000 to 3,000 mg of DLPA in the midafternoon with a carbohydrate, to replace the afternoon L-tyrosine dose. Start cautiously with the lower dosage of DLPA; if you feel "wired," lower the dose or stop taking DLPA. The nervous, excited feeling means that you probably don't need DLPA. A cautionary note is in order. If you are severely depressed, anxious, or agitated, be sure to consult with a holistic physician or naturopath while you're on this program. You should begin to feel better within two to three weeks. Once your depression has subsided, it's a good idea to stay on this protocol for six months and then gradually taper off.

There are rarely any adverse effects from L-tyrosine. DLPA, however, may cause slight changes in blood pressure. Occasionally, if the dosage is too high, people report headaches, insomnia, or irritability. If that happens to you, lessen the dosage until those side effects dissipate. I had to lower my intake of DLPA, because it made me agitated at higher levels. Remember that the drugs that are being used to treat depression may have mild to severe side effects. With DLPA it is possible to adjust the dose to relieve any side effects you experience.

This protocol has helped me by lowering my pain level significantly and elevating my mood. I now take these amino acids only in winter, during the cold, wet weather and long hours of darkness we experience in the Pacific Northwest, which tend to aggravate my pain and depression. Do not take DLPA if you are pregnant or diabetic, have phenylketonuria, or suffer high blood pressure or melanoma. You also should avoid DLPA if you are taking a monoamine oxidase inhibitor antidepressant.

DHEA

I believe that DHEA, scientifically named dehydro-3-epiandrosterone, holds great promise in treating lupus. It is a steroid precursor hormone that the body produces when we are young and healthy. As we age, however, we produce far less DHEA. A higher level of DHEA in our bodies has been found to lessen many age-related symptoms in both animal and human studies. Researchers have known since at least the 1980s that DHEA protects brain cells from Alzheimer disease and other senility-associated degenerative conditions.[15] Although DHEA is a steroid, it does not exhibit the strong hormonal influences of fully formed steroids, such as estrogen, testosterone, or progesterone; thus, those of us who are hormone sensitive may be able to take DHEA successfully.[16]

The DHEA in natural therapies is extracted from the South American yam and used in powdered form in capsules or as liquid plant extracts. Research points out that DHEA may be helpful in preventing and treating cardiovascular disease, high cholesterol, diabetes, obesity, cancer, Alzheimer's disease and other memory disturbances, and immune system disorders, including acquired immunodeficiency syndrome, chronic fatigue syndrome, and autoimmune disease. Blood serum DHEA levels have been documented to be lower than normal in patients with autoimmune disorders. Dr. Davis Lamson, a naturopath practicing in Kent, Washington, has found DHEA to be helpful in treating patients with two autoimmune diseases—ulcerative colitis and rheumatoid arthritis—as long as the initial DHEA blood and saliva tests show that the DHEA level is on the low side.[17]

Once I learned about DHEA, I was eager to find studies discussing its potential application in lupus. But I had to wait a number of years to find any such studies. Although this research is still in its infancy, it is encouraging. One vital study was performed on the New Zealand black mouse, which is subject to an autoimmune syndrome similar to SLE. Experiments have shown that when these animals are given DHEA, the autoimmune activity that can cause kidney failure and the hemolytic anemia that often accompanies SLE have been blocked. DHEA also increases the production of interleukin-2, a component of the immune system that is consistently low in those of us with lupus.[18]

Another study, this one conducted in the mid-1990s by James McGuire, M.D., chief of staff at Stanford University Hospital, shows promise for treating lupus patients with DHEA. A group of fifty-seven women with mild to moderate symptoms of lupus took 50 to 200 mg of oral DHEA every day for 3 to 12 months. About two-thirds reported some relief of their symptoms, including rashes, joint pain, headaches, and fatigue. Most of the women in the study stated that their ability to concentrate and their tolerance for exercise improved. "DHEA has the potential to be an important drug in [the treatment of] lupus, particularly because of its apparent ability to significantly reduce the need for steroids," reported Dr. McGuire. A subsequent year-long study determined the best dosage of DHEA for lupus patients.[19] It is important to remember that even though Dr. McGuire calls DHEA a "drug," it is a natural hormone.

There is more good news for lupus patients in the form of clinical trials to determine whether DHEA can help prevent and treat osteoporosis. Because many lupus patients are taking glucocorticoids, they are more vulnerable to osteoporosis than the average population. Glucocorticoids lower the levels of adrenal androgens, such as DHEA, which protect bone mass. In fact, prolonged administration of prednisone results in DHEA levels near zero.[20] New research is suggesting that some lupus patients taking DHEA can significantly lessen their glucocorticoid requirements over time, reducing their risk of osteoporosis.[21]

The news that DHEA may play a significant role in guarding against or reversing osteoporosis is hopeful for those of us with lupus. As we female lupus patients move into our menopausal and postmenopausal years, we need natural ways to protect our skeletal structures from fractures that could disable us permanently. Researchers know that DHEA levels diminish during menopause. In one study, the average plasma level of DHEA was 542 in premenopausal women, 197 in postmenopausal women, and only 126 in women whose ovaries had been removed surgically. In a group of women between the ages of 55 and 85 years, there was a significant correlation between serum levels of DHEA and the bone density of the vertebral spine. This study points out that women with higher levels of DHEA had more bone mass than those with lower DHEA levels.[22]

There is more research indicating the correlation between DHEA levels and strong bones. In one study of Belgian women, researchers discovered definite correlations between strong bones and adequate DHEA levels. A companion study illustrated the relationship between established osteoporosis and low DHEA levels. Although the DHEA levels declined with age in both groups of women, those women with osteoporosis consistently had lower DHEA levels at all ages. These studies support the use of DHEA in maintaining bone mass.[23] The difficulty with all of these studies is their female bias. It is highly likely that DHEA also can be of significant help to the approximately 10 percent of lupus patients who are male.

I began taking DHEA at the suggestion of an alternative physician in 1987, long before most American doctors were aware of it. A saliva test indicated that my DHEA levels were very low. Over the two years I took DHEA, I felt that I gained physical stamina from it, but I also came to suspect that it amplified my premenstrual symptoms. I think that a percentage of those of us with lupus are "allergic" to our own hormones—that is, our immune systems are attacking not only our organs but also the hormones in our blood. I stopped taking DHEA when I learned that it is a precursor to estrogen, to which I am allergic.

Since a recent bone scan has indicated that I have mild bone loss, I have started taking DHEA again at a low dose of 5 mg a day, hoping that it will increase my bone density. At this writing, there is no established minimum dose of DHEA for preventing osteoporosis. Those of us with lupus need to be concerned about our skeletal health for two reasons. Lupus can limit our physical activity severely over many years, and that inactivity can weaken our bone structure. Furthermore, research has established that there is a genetic predilection for osteoporosis. Those of us descended from people who have had osteoporosis need to be vigilant about trying to avoid its ravages if possible.

Because I believe that DHEA holds such great promise for lupus patients, I encourage you to give it a three- to six-month trial if you are not hormone sensitive and have mild to moderate lupus symptoms. If you have osteoporosis or are concerned about it, DHEA also may help you. Be sure to consult a naturopath or alternative physician about trying this natural agent, especially because there has been some recent concern about higher dosages of DHEA and potential side effects. If you cannot find a health professional who knows anything about DHEA, don't be discouraged. You can obtain copies through your public library of the articles I use as references in this chapter, or ask a librarian to help you locate information on DHEA and lupus. In addition, you can find articles and information on the Internet (see the resource section at the back of this book). Take the articles to your doctor and request that he or she read them so that you can discuss this treatment.

Using the Stanford study as a guideline, you can take 50 to 200 mg a day of DHEA safely. I would start with a much lower dosage—possibly 5 to 20 mg a day—and record how you feel. If you do not feel better in a few days, raise the dosage by 10-mg increments. Ideally, you will begin to feel better within two weeks, but do not be in a hurry. One of the standard rules of natural therapies is that they generally take significantly longer to work than pharmaceuticals. If you feel dizzy or depressed or start to retain fluid, you are most likely hormone sensitive and should stop taking DHEA. You can purchase DHEA at health food stores, but it is expensive to obtain doses that are high enough. A better approach may be to obtain DHEA in more concentrated form by prescription from compounding pharmacies (specialized pharmacies that prepare natural medicines from scratch).

Discovering and using these nine enormously helpful nutritional supplements over the years has helped me move close to the level of health I enjoyed before lupus entered my life. Over the long term, these supplements have lowered my levels of anxiety, depression, and pain. They also have increased my energy, strength, optimism, appetite, ability to endure heat and cold, my interest in life, and my belief that I ultimately will recover completely from lupus. I have no doubt that if you use two or three of these supplements, they will help you. Be cautioned, however, not to use more than a couple at a time or you won't be able to tell which one is helping. Talk with your alternative health care provider to determine which of these supplements you could start taking. It is very important for all of us with lupus to be proactive in searching for ways to minimize our lupus symptoms. Taking our power back helps us not only to feel better but also to believe that we have a life beyond lupus.

6

Healing Herbs

*Herbs have a unique spirit on the earth. We need to use them with
thanksgiving and wisdom.*

Linda Rector-Page, N.D., Ph.D.

Chamomile was the first herb I tried, hoping that it would relieve some of
the nervous system symptoms associated with my lupus. The effects of this
medicinal plant were immediate and dramatic. Drinking only one cup of
chamomile tea a day began to relieve my anxiety, confusion, and sleeplessness. Based on my positive response to chamomile, I was eager to explore
the healing potentials of other medicinal plants. And so I found myself
loading my camels once again, this time to travel in search of the best
sources of information on herbal healing.

As the camels lumbered slowly through the desert of mainstream health
care, I searched the horizon for a caravansary—a word derived from the
Persian for an inn on the trade route. This was where traders stopped to
water their camels and eat together inside the beautifully domed structures
of their walled encampments. Here they shared the knowledge of the goods
they were trading from all over Asia and the Middle East. Looking for the
traders in herbal traditions, I bivouacked at some fascinating caravansaries
on that journey. Talking with Europeans, Native Americans, Vietnamese,

Chinese, and East Indians gave me a grounding in cultures that have long traditions of using plants to heal illness. Studying with an American herbalist helped me search for specific herbs that might relieve lupus symptoms.

It is important to understand that when we use herbs for healing, we are part of a worldwide movement. In developing countries, 80 percent of the populations use plants as their primary medicines.[1] Doctors in many industrialized nations also practice herbal medicine. In the 1980s, for example, herbal preparations were prescribed as primary medicines by 30 to 40 percent of all medical doctors in France and Germany.[2] Although few American physicians currently prescribe herbs, consumers in the United States spent more than $12 billion in 1997 on natural supplements, possibly a third of which was on medicinal herbs.[3]

Why should we use healing plants? Put very simply, because they work. One great benefit of herbs is that they can be used along with other medicines with little danger of interactions. Another important advantage is that healing plants work at a cellular level, relieving the cause of disease, rather than just treating symptoms, as pharmaceuticals generally do. That means that you can stop taking a specific herb after a period of time, knowing that there is a good chance it has corrected the imbalance that has caused your illness. A third benefit of herbs is that if they are grown organically, they are environmentally clean, which helps both us and the planet. The final advantage is that you can grow many of these plants yourself. When you cultivate herbs and learn how to use them, you participate actively in your own healing.

There are three ways to take herbs for their maximum effect: as an infusion (or decoction), as a tincture (fluid extract) or solid extract, or as a whole herb. A tea, called an infusion or a decoction, is made from the dried herb. I prefer to use fresh herbs when they are available. Teas can be a better source of healing compounds than the powdered herb, because the hot water serves as a solvent in extracting the medicinal properties of the herb. But herb teas are weak in their action compared with tinctures, fluid extracts, and solid extracts.

Herbalists make tinctures by soaking the herb in an alcohol-and-water solvent for a specific period of time, to release the medicinal compounds.

Some herbs soak for only a few hours, some for many days, or even weeks. This process produces a concentrated tincture of the herb that we take in drops. We also can take herbs as solid extracts ground into powder and put into capsules. This powder is even more concentrated than the tincture and can be converted into a fluid extract or tincture in more concentrated form. Because they are exposed to air, which causes oxidation, powdered herbs are likely to be the least potent form of an herb.

Taking whole herbs gives us the best chance to heal. This is because researchers generally do not know which component of an herb has healing qualities. By using whole herbs, we benefit from the synergy among all the components of the plant. Lately, the word *standardized* is appearing on the labels of some herbal tinctures and capsules. It is important to note that this term does not guarantee the superiority of a product in any way, because at present there is no accepted definition of the word in this country.[4] Whether you are buying fresh or packaged herbs, be careful to purchase those that a trusted herbalist in your community recommends as being grown organically or not being overharvested, in the case of wild herbs.

My one difficulty with many herbal tinctures is the alcohol content, to which some of us with lupus are chemically sensitive. A naturopath suggested that I put the drops in very warm, not hot, water, which causes the alcohol to dissipate but retains the healing properties of the herb. If you are chemically sensitive, this approach will allow you to take herbal tinctures.

As a consumer of healing herbs, I have long been in a quandary about the kind of herbal preparations to buy. TCM tends to favor herbal formulas made from many herbs over the use of single herbs for the reason that, when used together in correct combinations, several herbs have greater healing capacity. In the early years of my illness, I purchased Chinese herbal formulas almost exclusively. I was always concerned, however, about the quality of the herbal preparations. I wondered whether the formulas were hygienically prepared and unadulterated. Had the medicinal plants been grown organically? Were endangered animals being killed for their body parts, which are added to some traditional Chinese herbal formulas?

I have never found satisfactory answers to these questions, but I do know that the medicinal plant industry in China is unregulated. Consequently, today I take very few herbs that are grown in China, preferring instead to take Chinese formulas made of the best-quality American herbs that are certified organic. This can be a difficult consumer choice, particularly if you need an herbal formula that is not compounded in this country. If you are having difficulty finding domestic herbal formulas that you think you need, discuss your concern with a naturopath or licensed TCM practitioner and follow his or her advice. For a more thorough discussion of Chinese medicinal herbs, see chapter 10, on lupus and TCM.

The following are the primary healing herbs that have helped limit or relieve many of my lupus symptoms. If you decide to try some of these herbs, be sure to consult a trained herbalist. If you are unable to access an herbalist, read at least two books on herbal therapies. Then start with very low doses of these plants to make sure you can tolerate them. Even though all of these herbs are nontoxic, you may still react to them, because they can be very powerful in their actions. I take smaller quantities of herbs than is generally recommended by herbalists, because herbs contain plant chemicals, called phytochemicals, to which I may be chemically sensitive. Since herbs work in the individual cells, they affect healing more slowly than pharmaceuticals. Try to give herbs a three- to six-month trial so that you can adequately measure their effectiveness.

My own journey over the herbal terrain began with the three-thousand-year-old Chinese herbal tradition. I was told by both of the TCM practitioners who were treating my lupus that I had kidney and spleen deficiency. In the TCM system the spleen is very important, because it is considered a digestive organ. The Chinese healing tradition thinks of the spleen as a set of patterns controlling the whole digestive process, from the eating of food to the elimination of waste.

An herbal formula for treating deficient spleen and other symptoms accompanying SLE is called compounded *Astragalus,* or *Astragalus* supreme. It is based on a Chinese herbal formula, but the tincture is produced in the United States from domestically grown plants. It contains schisandra, *(Schisandra chinensis)*, Chinese astragalus root *(Astragalus membranaceus)*, and Chinese ligustrum berry *(Ligustrum lucidum)*. This formula is used to treat the breakdown of immune functions. I believe that it has been a great help to me by lowering the level of autoimmune attack in my body. It also has helped me handle all kinds of stress more effectively. The three plants in the compound are plant adaptogens, which means that they work by positively supporting the functions of our organs and glands.

Plant adaptogens also are called immunomodulators, herbs that help bolster resistance and resilience to stress, enabling the body to avert various problems and avoid collapse by adapting to external pressures. These herbs work in a holistic way to affect positively the tissue in our bodies that creates our immune response.[5] From my own experience, I am convinced that one of the best holistic treatments for lupus lies in using these immunomodulators. They not only stimulate a weak immune system but also may calm down an overactive immune response, such as we experience with lupus.

The immunomodulators have the amazing ability to balance the body's functions. For example, if there is a hyperstate, some of these immunomodulating herbs can curb that effect. On the other hand, if there is sluggishness in the body, these herbs have a heightening effect. This action baffles allopathic pharmacologists, but it doesn't surprise experienced herbalists.[6] Specific to SLE, herb researchers think that immunomodulators may stimulate T suppressor cell function and thereby reduce immune resistance or lower the level of autoimmune response.[7] In other words, these plants may be able to calm our overactive immune systems, thereby lessening our level of autoimmune response.

Schisandra has been used in Asia since before the time of Christ for treating conditions of the spleen. It can be used effectively if you are recovering from illness or have depressed adrenal gland function as the result of stress. An added benefit of schisandra is that it helps the liver. In one test of 102 patients with infectious hepatitis, a cure rate of 76 percent was noted when patients ate powdered schisandra fruit over an extended period of time.[8] Overall, it has helped me feel stronger. If you are interested in trying this herb separately from the compounded astragalus formula, start with a very dilute mixture to make sure you can tolerate it. The usual dose is 6 to 9 g in a decoction, or you can eat dried schisandra fruits, which are available at Asian pharmacies and are delicious.[9] It is also available in pill form as a Chinese herbal preparation.

Astragalus helps balance the immune response, enabling it to be more flexible in the face of disease. Although it has some antiviral activity, the main effect of astragalus is to enhance interferon production and secretion. Recent research has shown that astragalus can intensify the activity of certain white blood cells, stimulate pituitary–adrenal cortical activity, and restore depleted red blood cell formation in bone marrow. It is an ideal remedy for many of us who are "immunocompromised."[10] Besides taking astragalus in tincture form, you also can make a tea from 1 to 4 g of the dried root and drink it three times a day, or take the powdered extract in capsule form at a strength of 200 to 500 mg three times a day.

Ligustrum, which is also part of the compounded astragalus formula, nourishes and tones the liver and kidneys. It has a rejuvenative action and specifically treats dizziness and tinnitus. Start with a very small dose to establish whether you can tolerate the formula. Then take 30 to 40 drops of the tincture three to five times daily in a small amount of warm water. If you are sensitive to the alcohol in this tincture, put the drops in a cup of very warm water, wait two minutes while the heat dissipates the alcohol, and then drink. Do not expect quick results. You will gain the most benefit from this formula by using it six months or longer. Don't use this compound if you are experiencing severe cold or flu symptoms.

Because lupus is a stress-sensitive illness, many of us with the disease need an enhanced ability to tolerate stress. We can start by minimizing the stress in our lives as much as possible. Then we can use herbs to help us tolerate the remaining stress more successfully. An important plant for protecting us against stress is another immunomodulator called ashwaganda (Withania somnifera: Solanaceae). An ayurvedic herb well known in India, it is an excellent strengthening tonic. I used this herb before I found the compounded astragalus and believe it strengthened me both physically and mentally. Ashwaganda is safe and effective and is not overstimulating. In fact, it promotes sound sleep and can treat arthritis and weakness of the mind. It also helps with joint and nerve pain and general convalescence.[11] An added benefit of ashwaganda is that it is less expensive than the various types of ginseng. You can find it in the ayurvedic herbal section of your health food store. Start with a very low dose to make sure you can tolerate it and then build up to the dosage recommended on the label. Give ashwaganda a good two-month trial to assess its benefits for you.

Another herb called gotu kola *(Centella asiatica)*, also has healing potential for lupus patients. A perennial plant native to India, China, Indonesia, Australia, the South Pacific, and southern and central Africa, it has been used in India since prehistoric times and is still used in the ayurvedic tradition to treat such skin conditions as eczema, psoriasis, and varicose ulcers. If you are experiencing extreme fatigue from lupus, this herb may be able to help. Gotu kola has been a great help to me in improving my ability to think clearly and express myself succinctly. Cognitive problems, such as the inability to read and recall what you've read, to think clearly from the first phase to subsequent phases of a problem, or to recall specific words and names, all can be improved greatly by gotu kola's specific actions. It is a stimulant to the central nervous system and is recommended by herbalists to improve memory and treat fatigue. Of particular importance to lupus patients is that gotu kola can enhance the development and maintenance of blood vessels supplying connective tissue, thereby helping to cleanse the connective tissue.[12] Take 10 to 20 ml per day of tincture or drink a tea made from 2 to 4 g of the crude dried plant leaves.

Another helpful ancient plant for treating cognitive problems is ginkgo *(Ginkgo biloba)*. Although the Chinese traditionally have used ginkgo as an antimicrobial and antitubercular agent, new research has shown that it also increases cardiovascular circulation, cerebral circulation, and brain function. It can treat vertigo, impairment of memory and ability to concentrate, and diminished intellectual capacity that result from insufficient circulation. Ginkgo may provoke stomach problems, so start with a very low dose. The standard dose is 40 mg of the dried herb in a tablet taken three times a day. I take a formula containing ginkgo, gotu kola, Siberian ginseng, schisandra, and ginger, which is helping me maintain enough mental clarity to write this book!

One of the most effective herbs I've taken is garlic *(Allium sativum)*. Its ability to heal the body amazes me. I first began taking garlic for stomach problems and found that it helped some of my other symptoms as well. It works as a preventive for most infectious conditions. I have not had a cold or the flu since I began taking garlic two years ago. Before then, I experienced two illnesses two winters in a row that seemed to approach pneumonia in their severity. Garlic encourages the growth of beneficial bacteria in the intestines while killing many pathogenic organisms in the intestinal tract. It is well known that garlic lowers cholesterol levels; it is less well known that garlic also can balance blood glucose levels. I used to get frantically hungry between meals, but since I began including garlic in my diet I no longer have that "hollow stomach" feeling.

All of us with lupus should eat garlic every day. If you can manage fresh garlic, eat one clove three times a day or put plenty of it in your cooked dishes. You can make a healthful garlic broth by taking three cups of vegetable broth made from one of the recipes in chapter 4 and adding one tablespoon of olive oil, one-half bay leaf, a pinch of dried sage, half a bulb or more of peeled, chopped garlic, one-eighth teaspoon dried thyme, and salt to taste. Bring to a boil, reduce heat, cover, and simmer for thirty minutes. Sip this broth or make thicker soups from it by adding vegetables. If you can't manage fresh garlic, take garlic oil or aged garlic in capsules. I took six capsules of garlic a day for six months and now take three capsules a day as a maintenance dose. Each capsule contains 300 mg of garlic extract. You can take a high dose of three capsules three times a day to stop an infection.

The nervine herbs are a group of plants that can help all of us with lupus. These herbs work to calm the nervous system and have many other actions as well. Chamomile *(Matricaria recutita)* is probably the most widely used relaxing nervine herb in the Western world. This plant helped me when I became ill in Turkey with an undiagnosable illness. In Turkey, pharmacists are trained in ancient herbal remedies as well as modern pharmaceuticals. I quickly learned to consult a Turkish pharmacist whenever I experienced physical symptoms, and my neighborhood pharmacist suggested chamomile to help calm my nerves and help me sleep. The dried chamomile flowers I brought home from the pharmacy, when steeped in hot water, imparted a lovely pink hue. I drank the tea three times a day, becoming calmer and more focused within one day. Years later, when I was suffering from severe stomach distress and ulcers, I went to our local bulk herb shop in Olympia, Washington, for help and came home once again with chamomile, which calmed my stomach and my general nervousness.

Chamomile is especially applicable to digestive problems produced by anxiety and tension, such as gas, colic pains, and even ulcers. It also can treat insomnia, anxiety, menopausal depression, loss of appetite, migraine, motion sickness, and vertigo. Chamomile is a mild antimicrobial. Breathing the steam of chamomile will treat inflamed sinus and lung membranes and remove excess mucus. It is best to use chamomile as a tea. Put two teaspoons of the dried plant in a cup of hot water, let it steep, and drink the tea three times a day. You can also take a tincture dosage of 1 to 4 ml three times a day.

There are three other nervine herbs that can help us be more calm and happy. Lavender *(Lavandula officinalis)* is one of these herbs. I have always loved the scent of lavender, and until I began studying herbal therapies, didn't realize that lavender can be taken internally to gain the full benefit of its many healing properties, particularly for those of us with nervous system difficulties. Lavender can alleviate stress headaches and lessen nervous exhaustion. Although I have not taken lavender internally, I often carry a tiny bottle of lavender essential oil with me, since I have discovered that breathing its vapors stops my headaches and calms me in stressful situations. Lavender also helps promote good sleep. Make a tea of one teaspoon of the dried herb to one cup of hot water and drink it three times a day. A cautionary note is that the oil of lavender should be used only externally.

Another helpful nervine herb is rosemary *(Rosmarinus officinalis)*. We have enjoyed adding rosemary to many of our casseroles over the years and hadn't realized it has healing effects. As a circulatory and nervine stimulant, it can smooth out our digestive processes and, like lavender, can treat headache and mild depression. Make an infusion of one to two tea-spoonsful of the dried herb and drink three times a day. The oil of rose-mary can be used to treat sciatica, neuralgia, and even premature baldness, by applying it to your skin.

The final nervine herb that offers potential for those of us with lupus is valerian *(Valeriana officinalis)*. The naturopath I was seeing prescribed valerian early in my illness for my extreme anxiety. I found that valerian relieved much of my anxiety and relaxed me physically, but I was somewhat groggy in the mornings, which can be a side effect of this plant. In addition to calming anxiety, valerian can be effective in banishing muscle tension, indigestion, and mild pain. Valerian also is used around the world as a relax-ing remedy for hypertension and stress-related heart problems. If you are suffering from anxiety, the dose of valerian has to be sufficiently high to be effective. The tincture dosage is from 2.5 to 5 ml (one-half to one teaspoon) to as much as 10 ml (two teaspoons). For extreme stress, you can repeat a single dose of one teaspoonful two or three times at short intervals.[13]

A small amount of valerian can gently slip you into sleep. It also can be mixed with passionflower for insomnia. Mix equal parts of the two tinc-tures and take 5 to 15 ml thirty minutes before retiring.[14] If you want to experiment with valerian, start with a very low dose, about one-fourth tea-spoon of the tincture. If it helps you and you do not experience side effects, you can raise the dose to two teaspoons of tincture, depending on the severity of your symptoms. This herb may take a number of weeks to become effective, and it will not work for the treatment of acute insomnia. Do not take valerian if you are using prescription antidepressants or anxi-olytics, such as Valium (diazepam), or in combination with alcohol or other depressant drugs.

St. John's wort *(Hypericum perforatum),* can be an effective treatment for mild to moderate depression. It is a medicinal herb that grows wild in many parts of the country. This herb has been a great help in relieving my depression without side effects. The documented clinical evidence from Europe of the healing qualities of St. John's wort is impressive. According to these reports, this plant is similar in its action to antidepressant drugs. If you want to discuss the clinically established effects of St. John's wort with your medical doctor, you can quote from the research that states:

> It inhibits the synaptosomal uptake of noradrenaline and serotonin and also inhibits GABA re-uptake. The crude extract inhibits MAO-A and MAO-B enzymatic activity. The extract has dopaminergic activity, similar to the drug bupropion [Zyban]. A phytochemical compound found in St. John's wort called hyperforium significantly contributes to the anti-depressant activity. Hypericum extract also causes an upregulation of central serotonergic receptors which is consistent with the mechanism of action of some synthetic anti-depressant drugs.[15]

There has been some discussion about whether St. John's wort causes photosensitivity to ultraviolet A and B light rays. This is important for those of us with lupus, because we tend to be photosensitive. European doctors who prescribe this herb suggest that it is best to stay away from fluorescent lighting while taking St. John's wort, but normal exposure to sun shouldn't cause photosensitivity in healthy people.[16] If you have lupus, however, you should stay completely out of the sun while taking St. John's wort. Follow the directions on the label. Do not take the herb if you are taking prescription antidepressants.

Another group of medicinal plants that holds great promise for those of us with digestive problems are the carminative herbs—those that relieve digestive gas and bloating. Volatile oils in these plants stimulate the digestive system to work properly. Peppermint (Mentha piperita), is one helpful carminative herb. When we purchased our rural property some years ago, we were delighted to inherit a small, aromatic, and vigorous peppermint garden, planted by the little girls whose family previously lived there. Over the ensuing years, I have enjoyed harvesting small quantities of the leaves, steeping them, and sipping peppermint tea during the day. Medicinally, peppermint is an ancient treatment for influenza and colds and has nervine properties that control anxiety. The oil from these wonderful leaves can allay nausea and also stimulate bile and the flow of digestive juices. If you have stomach problems, do try peppermint. You can make a tea of one teaspoon of the dried herb or one tablespoon of the fresh herb and drink it three times a day. Or take 1 to 2 ml of the tincture three times a day.

Fennel *(Foeniculum vulgare),* another carminative herb, can greatly relieve stomach and intestinal distress as well as stimulate the digestion. Specifically, it relieves flatulence. It also can ease bronchitis and calm coughs. The oil of fennel can be applied externally to soothe rheumatic and muscular pain. Make a tea of one to two teaspoonsful and drink it three times a day, or take 1 to 2 ml of the tincture three times a day.

Many people find that ginger *(Zingiber officinale)* is helpful. This plant has been used worldwide for a very long time for stimulating the appetite. Its widespread use is due not only to its wonderful flavor but also to its antioxidant and antimicrobial properties. It can treat fevers and may mitigate an ongoing low-grade fever that can be a lupus symptom. In ayurvedic medicine, ginger has been used for thousands of years as an effective treatment for digestive problems. In our family, we enjoy not only drinking ginger tea but also eating tiny bits of candied ginger that come in lovely green pottery "ginger jars." You can make a tea of one teaspoon of freshly grated or powdered ginger root to one cup of water whenever you feel the need for its effects.

Slippery elm *(Ulmus fulva)* has helped me with stomach and intestinal problems. The inner bark of the slippery elm tree is ground into powder. This herb calms the stomach and encourages bowel movements, which are important for moving toxins out of the body rapidly. Working as a soothing demulcent, it is a perfect treatment for sensitive, inflamed mucous membrane linings of the stomach, duodenum, and intestinal tract. Because it has nutritive value, slippery elm often is used as a food during convalescence, since it is gentle and easily assimilated. I take it two ways. Sometimes I mix a tablespoon in a glass of water and drink it. At other times I make a gruel using only enough water to achieve a to pudding consistency. If it's a bit tasteless, you can add a little brown rice syrup. For a drink, mix one part powdered bark to eight parts water. Bring to a boil and simmer gently for ten to fifteen minutes. Drink half a cup three times a day.

I believe that ginseng holds promise for relieving some lupus symptoms. Many varieties of ginseng have been used in Asia throughout history. Researchers think that ginseng has been used for two thousand to four thousand years in China. There are numerous accounts of medicinal ginseng written by Chinese herbalists during the Han dynasty of 206 B.C. to A.D. 220, based on much earlier writings. The Taoist philosopher, Lao-tzu wrote about the benefits of this herb in approximately 550 B.C.

The various types of ginseng are so popular in Asia today, and the supply is so depleted from overharvesting, that Hong Kong ginseng dealers now engage in a highly competitive search of the West Coast, Wisconsin, and Canada for the prized ginseng roots. Once the roots are harvested here, they are kiln-dried in the autumn and air-freighted to Hong Kong for distribution all over Asia. In China many people start taking ginseng by age forty to slow aging and prevent illness. The Chinese traditionally have believed that ginseng can fight cancer, slow aging, strengthen digestion, protect against heart attack and other sudden illness, and lower high blood pressure, among other benefits. They take ginseng in capsules, tablets, candy, wine, chewing gum, and cooked in their food.

These plants are adaptogens that can nourish organs and tissues to prevent disease. Ginseng will not cure, but it will support and balance. A TCM practitioner will try to determine which imbalances are present in your body and then pick one of the varieties of ginseng to add to an herbal formula to support the fine-tuning of your bodily functions.[17] Based on my experience, I believe that there is potential help for lupus patients among the various kinds of ginseng. All of them are stimulants, some far stronger than others. Because these are powerful herbs, you should not self-administer; instead, you will need to work closely with an herbalist, a naturopath who is well schooled in the use of herbs, or a TCM practitioner.

During the worst years of my lupus I was weak and cold, had no energy, and became socially withdrawn because involvement with people was so exhausting. The first TCM practitioner I saw recommended red *Panax* ginseng to alleviate fatigue, stimulate circulation, stop heart palpitations, and calm anxiety. I took the red ginseng combined in a formula with the spleen-tonifying herb astragalus for one month. Red *Panax* ginseng has the power to improve mental fatigue, physical fatigue, sleep problems, appetite, digestion, immune function, and the shortness of breath of asthma. It also can rebalance psychological disturbances.[18]

This form of ginseng helped me feel stronger, but the TCM practitioner thought it was too powerful for me and switched me to white *Panax* ginseng, the mildest of the Asian ginsengs. This, combined with ginger or licorice, can help support our chi, which the Chinese believe is our life force. I took this formula for two more months, slowly feeling physically and mentally more stable. It is important not to take the ginsengs for too long, because even the milder ones are stimulants.

If you have mild lupus, are less than thirty-five years old, and are not cold or extremely debilitated, another form of ginseng, called American ginseng, may be appropriate for you. It is the most balanced of the *Panax* ginsengs and can nourish the yin—the soft, female energy—by supporting the adrenals, regulating the basic metabolism, increasing salivation, and clearing heat. It also can treat mental exhaustion and poor appetite.

Native Americans were using American ginseng long before Europeans arrived. The Cherokees traditionally used it for short-windedness, rheumatism, and bad appetite and as a cure for severe illness when all other treatments failed. The Iroquois used it to cure laziness and to heal tuberculosis.[19] Talk with your holistic health care provider to decide whether this ginseng might help you. Try to get woods-grown American ginseng because it is more effective than the commercially grown plant. Take it in a capsule or a tincture and start with low doses.

If you have very mild to mild lupus or if you are in remission from lupus, the herb eleuthero *(Eleutherococcus senticosus)*, also called Siberian ginseng, may be a good tonic for you. I occasionally take Siberian ginseng for one month as a tonic. It is more neutral than the *Panax* ginsengs, and not as stimulating, and it can strengthen you through its support of spleen and kidney function. It also can help you deal with stress by supporting your adrenal function, and it will fortify your immune response. Eleuthero can even help the muscles utilize oxygen and energy stores more efficiently. It does not induce estrogen and testosterone effects as the *Panax* ginsengs do, and so you can take it even if you are hormone sensitive. It stimulates the pituitary gland, however, which helps regulate all the hormonal functions of the body. I prefer to take the tincture form of Siberian ginseng, two full droppers at a time, one in the morning and another in the evening.[20] Start with only one full dropper per day and work up over five to six days to the full dose. If you have more than a mild case of lupus, do not take Siberian ginseng for more than three months at a time.

There is one final important point about herbal therapy for lupus patients. Because those of us with lupus have overactive immune systems that are attacking our own tissue, it would seem wise to avoid the immunostimulating herbs that could cause the immune system to become even more overactive. On the other hand, taking an immune-enhancing herb during a short period of infection would still be appropriate for a lupus patient because the immune system is basically compromised. I have been helped greatly by taking echinacea, nettle, and garlic in high doses for three days to two weeks when I've been ill with colds or the flu. But I cannot tolerate goldenseal, and I have avoided the other immunostimulating herbs because my immune system has been fighting abnormally hard for so long. Additional herbs that can help fight short-term infections include burdock, cleavers, sarsaparilla, yellow dock, calendula, myrrh, onion, western hemlock, and wild indigo. Be aware that as a lupus patient you should not take these herbs for longer than two weeks at a time.

In addition to the herbs I've mentioned in this chapter, there are seven other primary herbs that may be used by naturopaths for treating lupus. Although I have not used these herbs, I list them here to give you additional healing plants to discuss with your holistic care provider. They are *Berberis vulgaris, Chimaphila umbellata, Hydrangea arborescens, Juniper communis, Thuja occidentalis, Avena sativa,* and *Althea officinalis.*[21–23] Other nutritive and tonic herbs that may relieve lupus symptoms are *Medicago sativa, Rumex officinalis, Taraxacum officinale,* and *Urtica dioica.*[24]

Many of the herbs described in this chapter have helped me regain my health. Today we grow medicinal herbs in our garden that we harvest, dry, and prepare as tonics. Our family intends to go on learning about herbs and using them to stay healthy. Herbs provide a relatively inexpensive alternative to frequent doctors' appointments and allow us to take a proactive role in improving our health. If you are a gardener and live in a warm, sunny climate, you can grow many healing herbs yourself, harvesting them and using them in teas and tinctures as an inexpensive way to support your health. If you are physically unable to garden, perhaps a friend or relative would agree to grow medicinal herbs for you. Whichever approach you decide to take, you are likely to experience a lessening of many of your lupus symptoms by using these wonderful healing plants.

7

Beneficial Fats and Oils

Adding electron-rich, highly unsaturated fats to our diets is critically important to oxygenate our bodies, protecting us from disease.

Johanna Budwig, M.D.

The kind of fat we eat is crucial to good health. In fact, if we are ill, the kind of fat we include in our meals may affect whether we stay chronically ill or begin healing. There are even nutritionists who say that the quality of the fat we put in our mouths may be instrumental in making us sick in the first place. The biochemist Udo Erasmus, in his book *Fats and Oils*, discusses the critical role proper fat metabolism plays in keeping us healthy. "Deranged fat metabolism lies at the root of most degenerative disease. This derangement may be caused by too much of the wrong kinds of fat in our diet, too much total fat, or deficiency of the right kind of fats."[1] In this chapter, we explore the role beneficial fats play in optimum health. More specifically, I discuss my own experience with changing the types of fats I eat, and the resulting alleviation of my lupus symptoms. First, let's learn a bit about fats that are not good for us.

THE DAMAGING OMEGA-6 FATS

The two types of omega-6 fats and oils are saturated fat and polyunsaturated oils. Those of us with lupus need to think about how much of these fats and oils we eat, because each type of omega-6 fat is detrimental to health. Let's examine the dangers of saturated fat first. This type of fat includes all animal fats, coconut oil, and palm oil. It stays solid at room temperature. Although we should not be eating this type of fat, it is difficult to avoid, because the American diet is literally saturated with saturated fats. When we eat Mom's apple pie made with a crust containing solid vegetable shortening or when we eat fatty red, pink or white meats, we are harming our body chemistry inestimably.

What damage do omega-6 saturated fats do to our bodies? These fats cause deranged fat metabolism and stimulate the liver to make low-density lipoprotein (LDL, or 'bad') cholesterol in such large quantities that our systems can't remove it all. The leftover LDL severely damages the arterial walls, leading to atherosclerosis, which restricts the cardiovascular system from performing efficiently. Thus, saturated fat dramatically increases the risk of coronary heart disease and premature death. Equally important to those of us with long-term chronic illness is that saturated fat causes arteriosclerosis, which restricts blood flow, reducing the supply of oxygen to our cells and thereby limiting the body's healing capacity.[2] Another negative effect of saturated fat is that it produces PGE_2, which causes pain and inflammation if present in the body at abnormally high levels.

I knew very little about dietary fats when I began my safari through nutritional research. After reading the current data on fats and oils and talking with alternative health practitioners about the role of fats in health, I now believe the saturated fat I ate before the onset of my lupus may have contributed to my illness in many ways, particularly by causing arteriosclerosis, which restricted oxygen flow to my cells. Many of us who grew up in the 1950s and 1960s ate huge quantities of saturated fat found in beef, pork, and chicken. Most of us also ate cakes and cookies made with butter and vegetable oils, as well as three glasses of whole milk a day and toast slathered with butter. In that era the general public was unaware of the dangerous health implications of eating saturated animal fat.

Surrounded by so much fat in the American diet, we have little chance to experience cultures where people do not eat animal fat. Perhaps a glimpse into such a culture can offer us some perspective. My own saturated fat diet changed radically in my early twenties when I went to East Africa with the Peace Corps. In northwestern Uganda, our diets included little animal protein and thus little saturated fat. Because we lived in a tsetse fly–infested area where hoofed animals rarely survived, meat was seldom available.

My meat and fat craving sometimes sent me bicycling through the brilliant equatorial sunrise to the tiny open-air market on Saturday mornings, hoping I might be lucky enough to find a chicken for sale. But only rarely did I find a bird I could take home for stewing. Eating this diet very low in fat and animal protein, I lost more than twenty pounds but maintained plenty of energy. Teaching seven hours a day and monitoring the two-hour evening study period at our secondary school, I still had the strength to cultivate and water a vegetable garden by hand, bicycle into the village on errands, and trek through the bush hoping to spot elephants, monkeys, and leopards. Even though I felt well, I also often felt hungry.

The people in my region were generally thin, muscular, and very strong. The women particularly seemed to have unlimited energy, working many hours a day through the heat on their small banana and coffee farms. Most of these rural people had less food than I had. They were fortunate to eat a bit of stewed chicken once a year, and that probably would have been for a holiday feast. They depended instead on boiled peanut sauce for their fat and protein, which they served over boiled plantain, called *matoke*. But many peasants were too poor to afford even peanut sauce.

With little to eat other than *matoke*, which is primarily carbohydrate, these people seemed malnourished to me. Although the Polish doctor in our village sometimes saw cases of malnutrition, he had an interesting observation about the general diet of the Ugandans in our region. If it weren't for the often deadly parasitic infestations that many of these people endured, the doctor told me they would have been among the strongest, healthiest populations he had seen anywhere in the world. This, he said, was precisely because they ate a plant-based diet. The doctor's perspective surprised me. How could it be, I wondered, that these people whom I regarded as underfed because they did not eat meat and fat, might, in fact, be some of the healthiest people alive? I vowed to start eating *matoke* right away, but I soon realized that I couldn't eat much of it without feeling bloated. And frustrating as it was, I still craved meat and fat.

Once in a while that craving was satisfied when an angel appeared at my door in the guise of an elderly man selling Nile perch wrapped in banana leaves. A tender, sweet-tasting fish, Nile perch would be considered a delicacy anywhere in the world. I hardly could contain my delight at the prospect of fish for dinner, but I was also concerned that the perch might be spoiled from being unprotected during the many hours this exhausted man had spent pedaling thirty miles through scorching heat from Lake Albert. I always bought the Nile perch, however, and risked eating it, knowing that I could become gravely ill. Hunger leads us to take risks.

On rare occasions I received a gift of enough fat and protein to last me a few days. Imagine my delight when Norwegian Peace Corps friends rattled up in their decrepit Volkswagen Beetle, producing from the little trunk a three-pound roast from a legally shot wildebeest. This was cause for celebration! Wildebeest is lean, flavorful, and tender. I set it to baking in short order on my little two-ring propane stove in a covered baking pan very much like a Dutch oven. Later, our joking and laughter echoed through the bush as we relished a rare dinner with enough food for all of us.

During those years in eastern Africa, I never would have believed that I would someday be writing about the dangers of saturated animal fats. Searching for enough food in the eastern African savanna, I welcomed any animal fat that found its way to my table. Even though my Ugandan students and neighbors were modeling eating more healthily, I did not understand fully that eating less fat and less food in general was good for me. The rice, fruits, fresh bread, small amounts of milk and yogurt, and small portions of fish and wild game that I ate were a much better diet than I had eaten traditionally. Today, by contrast, it is difficult to ignore the research on rats and mice that suggests that undereating may safeguard health and increase longevity.[3]

Far from welcoming animal fat to my table today, I now recognize the wisdom of drastically limiting our saturated fat intake or, better yet, banning it from our diets. Of all the saturated fats, beef fat is the greatest threat to health. Other natural sources of dangerous dietary fat are unskinned chicken, pork, lamb, duck, whole milk, cheese, butter, cream, and all packaged foods made with palm kernel oil. The unnatural sources of saturated fat include margarine, solid vegetable shortening, and all processed foods made with partially hydrogenated oils.

Although it may be difficult for us to stop eating saturated fat, it is important that we address this issue. We can start with small steps, such as eliminating bacon at breakfast and substituting a bit of nut butter for real butter on our toast. Then we can eliminate the traditional Sunday roast beef dinner and serve fresh baked fish instead. If we read labels on processed foods carefully for saturated fat content, we can avoid those foods. Cooking from scratch more often will give us control over the fat content of our meals. Serving dessert only once or twice a week can encourage our families to leave the table feeling satisfied without the huge fat content of desserts. I know families who eat dessert only once a month! These incremental steps can wean us away from the damaging saturated fats we eat, while helping us avoid the fat-withdrawal blues. Over the long term, following this plan gives us a good chance to lose weight, gain energy, and improve our family's health.

The polyunsaturates represent another category of omega-6 fats that are not good for us, except possibly in very small quantities. Although polyunsaturated oils were in favor into the 1980s, we now know that they can be harmful. "We chose the wrong fat," say the chairmen of major nutrition departments.[4] These oils include corn, soy, sesame, sunflower, safflower, peanut oil, cottonseed oil, and grapeseed oil. It is important to understand a bit about the chemistry of polyunsaturates and how they affect the body. Polyunsaturated oils are biochemically unstable. When they are processed with chemicals or heat, a process called hydrogenation, they form trans-fatty acids, which can be extremely toxic. These toxic compounds harm DNA and cell membranes, leaving us vulnerable to inflammation and degeneration of tissue. That fact suggests that these oils are particularly dangerous for those of us with lupus, because our illness involves tissue inflammation.

Even worse news about polyunsaturated oils comes from Andrew Weil, M.D., who believes that they may damage the regulatory machinery of the body, significantly compromising the healing system.[5] Heeding this strong warning, I regret having eaten safflower oil in the years when I was deeply ill, but the research at that time suggested that polyunsaturates were far better for us than saturated fats. I now suspect that safflower oil may have hindered my body's efforts to heal from lupus by increasing my toxicity.

Equally alarming is the emerging research that indicates that polyunsaturated fat raises the risk of cancer by 69 percent. The Western diet includes up to twenty times as many omega-6 as the "good" omega-3 fatty acids, or a 20:1 ratio. If we are eating healthily, that ratio should be only about 4:1. Dean Ornish, M.D., an expert on cardio-nutrition (the best way to eat for a healthy heart), states that American women are eating five hundred times the amount of omega-6 that is considered healthy.[6]

There is another point of view, however, about the polyunsaturated oils. Later in this chapter, the polyunsaturates are described as containing essential fatty acids, which we need to stay healthy. For this reason, small quantities of safflower oil, for example, that has not been subjected to chemicals or heat may benefit us. The clinical research is still not definitive on the subject of omega-6 polyunsaturates. However, there seem to be enough indicators that these oils are dangerous when processed to suggest that lupus patients should avoid them.

THE HELPFUL OMEGA-9 FATS

After reading this information on the "bad" fats and oils, you're sure to be wondering whether there is any oil left that you can eat. You'll be happy to know that there is a third group of fats, the omega-9 monounsaturates, that we can eat in moderation, without worrying that they will harm us. In fact, the unrefined monounsaturated fats seem to benefit us. Of the six oils—

olive, canola, peanut, almond, avocado, and apricot kernel—olive is thought to be the best for us.

Briefly exploring a society where olive oil is used as a dietary staple may help us learn about the benefits of monounsaturated oils. Twenty years ago I had the good fortune to live in an "olive culture" for a time and was able to experience the health benefits of olives and olive oil. The Turkish family with whom I lived in Istanbul ate only unrefined olive oil, with its slightly heavier texture and fruity taste. We also ate lamb and chicken, containing saturated fat but in much smaller quantities than I had eaten in the United States. Our meals were mainly vegetarian, with huge amounts of rice, garbanzo beans, steamed or sautéed vegetables, dried fruits, nuts, and yogurt. We cooked with olive oil and ate a lot of whole olives. The breakfast menu nearly every morning comprised black olives with fresh rye bread and feta cheese. Dinner consisted of a number of steamed or sautéed vegetable dishes served with olive oil.

During trips to southern Turkey, we enjoyed long walks through groves of olive trees, their leathery leaves flashing green and silver in the wind. The bark of the olive trees was dark and craggy, suggesting that they were an ancient species whose genetic forebear witnessed the Greek and Roman legions on the march. Archaeological evidence verifies that edible olive tree orchards existed on the island of Crete as early as 3500 B.C. Over time they came to be cultivated in all the countries bordering the Mediterranean. Olive trees can survive in arid regions, producing their dark, chewy fruit with little moisture. Because they are quite disease resistant, olive trees need few, if any, chemical sprays to produce a crop. For that reason, we can safely assume that most olives and olive oil we buy are organically grown.

One of my first impressions of the Turkish people was that they generally seemed to be slender and energetic. I attributed that to the fact that everyone walked a great deal—even in the cities—at a very fast pace. I lost weight, too, believing that it was because I walked so much in Istanbul. At the end of many tiring days of teaching, I watched disconsolately as yet another overcrowded, top-heavy bus pulled away from the curb, leaving me stranded once again, to walk long distances through narrow cobbled streets to our apartment overlooking the Bosporus straits.

Today I know that the physical activity of the Turkish people, coupled with their high intake of vegetables, rice, grains, and olive oil keeps them slender, gives them energy, and increases their fat metabolism, thus guarding their health. Formal research is beginning to indicate that Mediterranean peoples have lower rates of cardiovascular and degenerative disease than populations who do not eat olive oil.

After many months of eating olive oil, I remember noticing that in addition to losing weight, my upper back muscles did not seem to spasm and ache as much, my skin was softer, and I had more energy. Nutritional studies are showing that we seem to be able to metabolize olive oil quite well. The best olive oil is called *extra virgin,* which is the first pressing and is not extracted with heat or chemicals. Instead, it is produced by applying mechanical pressure to the olives and should be labeled *expeller pressed.*

Olive oil has been an integral part of the meals we serve in our home for many years now. We have grown to prefer olive oil over other fats and now dribble olive oil on our potatoes, salads, and vegetable dishes. Baking remains a challenge, however, because many recipes call for butter or solid vegetable shortening. We substitute unsweetened applesauce for the oil in many recipes now, and we also bake with olive oil whenever possible. Recently we made an olive oil pie crust that was acceptable, though the texture was not as good as crust made with solid vegetable oil. But we're willing to compromise to safeguard our health. Most experts agree that the best oils for cooking are canola and olive oil, because these oils are composed primarily of oleic acid, a monounsaturated oil that is more resistant to the damaging effects of heat and light, compared with such highly polyunsaturated oils as corn and safflower.[7]

If you decide to replace butter, margarine, and vegetable oils with omega-9 monounsaturated oils—particularly olive oil—you may give yourself an advantage in improving your health. Be aware, though, that you will need to commit to this dietary change for the rest of your life to alter your body chemistry enough to support the healing process.

THE BENEFICIAL OMEGA-3 OILS

Another category of oils that bestows great health-enhancing benefits are the omega-3 oils. These contain essential fatty acids, or EFAs, which are found in oil made from the seeds of flax, walnut, pumpkin, and soybeans. They also are present in the oil of some fatty fish. Two of the most important EFAs are eicosapentaenoic acid (EPA) and docosahexaenoic acid (DHA), which are present in specific kinds of fish oil.

EPA AND DHA

We need these fatty acids in our diets to help protect us against cancer. EPA and DHA also protect us against degenerative disease by enhancing oxygen use in our cells. Another critical role EFAs play in safeguarding our health is strengthening the tissues of our adrenal glands, retinas, sex glands, brain cells, and inner ears. We can produce our own EFAs if we are healthy, but if we have degenerative disease, our bodies are likely to lose that capacity.

Assuming that many of us with lupus have lost the ability to produce EFAs, it becomes important to include them in our diets. Cold-water, fatty fish is a great addition to our meals and can supply us with sufficient EPA and DHA. You'll be happy to learn, as I was, that cold-water, fatty fish do not contain saturated fat. When I was growing up on the Pacific Northwest coast, my family ate lots of Pacific ocean salmon brought to our home by my grandfather's Native American friends. My grandmother often talked about how healthy she thought the tribe's diet was. Now we know why. In their highly unsaturated state, EPA and DHA not only strengthen the tissues but also help disperse globules of saturated fatty acids, which tend to stick together. This affords great support in keeping the arteries unplugged and blood platelets from sticking together and in lowering blood pressure significantly.[8] It is important to note this remarkable ability of EPA and DHA to help us recover from some of the damage saturated fats may have done to our bodies.

The best fish for supplying EFAs are high-fat, cold-water fish, such as trout, salmon, mackerel, sardines, halibut, and eel. Holistic nutritionists suggest that we eat this type of beneficial fish at least twice a week. Low-fat fish, such as pike, carp, haddock, and tuna, also contain EPA and DHA but in much smaller amounts. Fresh, free-swimming fish are the best source of EFAs. If you are unable to obtain wild fish, fish-farmed, cold-water fish may be an alternative. They may be of a lower quality, however, because there can be spoilage problems with commercial fish foods. Frozen ocean fish provide EFAs of the lowest quality. If you are unable to eat fresh, cold-water, fatty fish or you think that you need higher doses of EPA and DHA than fresh fish can furnish, you should take fish oil capsules. Be sure to look for "molecularly distilled" fish oils. This will assure you that the pesticides, PCBs (polychlorinated biphenyls), and heavy metals have been removed from the fish oils through a steam-stripping process. Take 120 mg to 1,800 mg a day, in three divided doses just before each meal.[9]

LA and LNA

The EFAs linoleic acid (LA) and linolenic acid (LNA) also are essential to us. Experts believe deficiency of these fatty acids is widespread in the American population. Because we cannot produce LA and LNA in our bodies, we need to obtain them from eating specific kinds of oil. To understand their importance, let's look at the symptoms of LA and LNA deficiency. Without an adequate supply of LA, we may experience kidney degeneration, excessive thirst, chronic infections, arthritis, eczema, hair loss, and behavioral disturbances. Symptoms of LNA deficiency include vision impairment, learning problems, physical weakness, and tingling in the arms and legs.

The list of benefits researchers have compiled for LA and LNA is long. These EFAs can help those of us with chronic illness through their biochemical attraction to oxygen, which gives them amazing oxygen-carrying properties. They play an essential role in creating life energy from the foods we eat and moving that energy into our cells. If people are extremely deficient in LA, for example, they literally can die from lack of oxygen.

LA and LNA not only transport oxygen, but also hold oxygen in the cell membranes, where it protects our cells against viruses and bacteria. This is important for those of us with lupus, who may have enhanced susceptibility to infections. Those of us with general physical exhaustion can be helped by the added energy that LA and LNA can furnish us. Because I have had muscle pain with lupus, I have been heartened to learn about the benefits of LA and LNA in that regard. When we exercise, our muscles produce lactic acid. If the lactic acid does not leave the muscles, it causes pain. LA and LNA help the body convert lactic acid to water and carbon dioxide, which are easily cleared from the body. This lessens or eliminates muscle pain and fatigue.

These EFAs also can assist in creating prostaglandins. LA produces PGE_1, which is very important in helping avert heart attacks and strokes. PGE_1 also slows down cholesterol production. It prevents inflammation, regulates calcium metabolism, improves nerve function, and controls arthritis. It also may hinder cancer cell growth by regulating the rate at which cells divide. LNA produces PGE_3, which reduces platelet stickiness and thereby protects us from blood clots of the arteries and brain.

There is a particular reason that those of us with lupus need to have LA and LNA in our diets. At the end of their biochemical pathways through the body, these fatty acids become prostaglandins, which perform the very important role of enhancing the action of our T lymphocytes. We have learned that T lymphocytes, which are primary immune cells, generally are deficient in SLE and other autoimmune diseases. It would follow, then, that if we can increase the body's ability to make T lymphocytes, we may be able to alleviate lupus symptoms. More specifically, it is the T lymphocytes, or suppressor T cells, that stop the B cells from destroying our own tissue. Suppressor T-cell levels are always low in lupus patients.[10] It is possible that by eating sources of LA and LNA, we can create more prostaglandins, which in turn will raise our suppressor T-cell levels. That could help stop the immune system attacks on our own tissue.

How can we include LA and LNA in our diets? The richest source is flaxseed oil. Hemp oil, another excellent source, is now available in some health food stores in the United States. Soy oil and walnut oil are also excellent sources of these EFAs, but they may not be easy to find. Neither safflower oil nor sunflower oil contains any LNA, but they do contain LA.

Johanna Budwig, a German medical doctor, has devoted her life to the study of fats in the human diet. She is a brilliant researcher who has been nominated for the Nobel Prize in medicine. Dr. Budwig believes that much degenerative disease results from fatty acid deficiencies. Her research suggests that our saturated fat diets are killing us and that LA- and LNA-containing flaxseed oil is the key to correcting our dysfunctional fat metabolism. Dr. Budwig says that we need to eat a sulfur-containing protein food with the flaxseed oil to render the oil water soluble.[11] The best complement to flaxseed oil is sulfur-containing skim milk cottage cheese. She highly recommends a mixture of 100 g skim milk cottage cheese to 40 g flaxseed oil and 25 g skim milk. If you are sulfur sensitive, try reducing the amount of skim milk cottage cheese you eat with the flaxseed oil. You can also dribble fresh flaxseed oil on potatoes, vegetables, and salads.

The flaxseed oil we eat should be expeller pressed, and as unrefined as possible, kept in dark glass away from light, and refrigerated. It should not be used in cooking, since heat can affect its chemical composition. Healthy people can take two tablespoons of flaxseed oil a day. I am able to take only one teaspoon of flaxseed oil a day; any more seems to make me shaky. I believe this effect stems from the fact that my liver cannot metabolize much fat. Over the long term, however, I think that flaxseed oil has helped me by boosting my energy level, improving my symptoms of dry eye and dry mouth, relieving my eczema, and softening my skin. Try taking up to one tablespoon of this oil once daily or dividing the dose to accompany your three meals. It is somewhat expensive. If you are unable to take the oil because of the cost, you can eat the same quantity of flax seeds, which will still give you the benefit of the LA and LNA they contain. Soak the seeds in water for four to eight hours and strain. These seeds are slippery, so you need to chew them thoroughly to release the EFAs that can improve your health.[12]

The Benefits of GLA

Gamma linolenic acid, or GLA, also may benefit lupus patients by reducing pain level. Although our bodies theoretically can produce GLA from LA, inadequate diets, particularly high sugar consumption, interferes with this conversion. GLA produces the beneficial PGE_1 and PGE_3, which we learned earlier can help suppress pain in our bodies. It's important for lupus patients to know that steroids, such as prednisone, inhibit the beneficial effects of these prostaglandins. For this reason, it is possible that lupus patients with mild to moderate forms of the disease will benefit from a three-month trial of GLA, particularly if they are taking steroids. GLA will *not* help lupus patients who are taking more than small doses of steroids.[13]

We can get GLA from evening primrose oil, which is quite expensive. Borage oil, black currant oil, and spirulina microalgae also supply GLA and are less expensive. Oil of evening primrose has been used as a medicinal agent for a very long time. When the Pilgrims arrived in North America, they found Native Americans using this plant oil for healing external wounds and skin eruptions. They also took the oil internally for coughs and infections.[14]

Many studies have established the benefits of evening primrose oil. It can be effective in preventing liver damage from alcoholism, and it can lower blood pressure, decreasing the risk of strokes and heart attack. Because it raises the metabolic rate, evening primrose oil can enhance the burn-off of fat, helping overweight people lose unwanted pounds. In women it also relieves premenstrual breast pain, bloating, irritability, and depression, which can lead to aggressive behavior.[15] In laboratory tests, the oil of evening primrose has blocked the development of arthritis in animals.

Beyond pain suppression, there appear to be other possible therapeutic effects of evening primrose oil on autoimmune disease. Rheumatoid arthritis and diabetes are both considered to be autoimmune illnesses. In recent studies, evening primrose oil has reversed moderate cases of rheumatoid arthritis.[16] In a clinical trial in 1993, it was shown that GLA supplementation can improve nerve function in diabetic patients and prevent diabetic nerve disease. The dose used in the trial was small—only 240 to 480 mg of GLA per day.[17] This information on GLA and diabetes is valuable, because allopathic physicians often administer high doses of steroids to lupus patients and steroids may cause diabetes. It is known that multiple sclerosis, an autoimmune condition that affects the sheaths of the nerves, can result from a prostaglandin imbalance. In Britain, oil of evening primrose is used by multiple sclerosis patients to slow down or stop the deterioration of their condition, because GLA can raise the level of beneficial PGE$_1$.[18]

Although I have been unable to locate specific research examining the use of GLA to treat SLE, my own experience may lead you to take supplements of this fatty acid, to see whether it will help relieve some of your lupus symptoms. In the years before I knew about flaxseed oil, I was eating safflower oil and supplementing with evening primrose oil to try to relieve some of my symptoms. The butterfly rash on my cheek as well as the severe rashes I had around my eyes and on my arms, hips, stomach, and legs all cleared up. My premenstrual symptoms dissipated, and I slowly developed more energy. I also felt the pain in my hands, hips, back, shoulders, neck, and head subside, though it did not vanish altogether. Taking evening primrose and flaxseed oil has helped alleviate many of my symptoms significantly.[19]

It is possible that evening primrose oil can help us, but we need to be aware that GLA is the subject of some controversy. Researchers still are not able to determine the absolute safety of GLA. There is evidence that over a period of time, GLA will cause damage by increasing arachidonic acid (unsaturated fatty acid) levels in the tissues. GLA also may lessen tissue levels of EPA, the beneficial fatty acid we spoke of earlier, which is found in cold-water fatty fish and in flaxseed oil. Some researchers believe that oils like safflower and soy, which contain high levels of linoleic acid, may provide as much benefit as GLA products at a fraction of the cost.[20] If that is the case, possibly the only people who need GLA are those who cannot convert linoleic acid to GLA. Otherwise, taking flaxseed oil can give us both the EPA and linoleic conversion to GLA that we need for prostaglandin production.

If you are able to afford to supplement with a GLA product, such as evening primrose oil or borage oil, you may want to give it a three-month trial. It will take at least that long for your body chemistry to correct enough to notice an amelioration in your symptoms. It is important that you take zinc, vitamin C, and vitamins B_3 and B_6 with whichever GLA oil you choose. These supplements are necessary to help your body convert the GLA to PGE_1. Vitamins E and A are also crucial for the body to keep EFAs intact and allow them to be metabolized properly. Since GLA will affect your metabolism, be aware that you may feel slightly worse for the first week or two, but you should begin to feel better within two to three weeks. If you continue to feel worse, stop taking the GLA supplement.

Take four to six capsules of GLA-containing oil twice a day before meals. When your symptoms improve, cut back to three capsules twice a day. A maintenance dose is three capsules per day.[21] If GLA supplementation does nothing, try flaxseed oil supplementation instead, which will have a good chance of helping you feel better if you give it a long enough trial.

I feel much better since I changed the types of fat in my diet. I now take a product that is a mixture of cold-pressed flaxseed oil, sunflower oil, sesame oil, evening primrose oil, rice germ oil, oat germ oil, and bran oil, for a combination of omega-3, omega-6, and omega-9 fatty acids. Here are some final suggestions for changing the quality and quantity of fat in your diet.

- Eat very little or no animal protein. Instead, eat large amounts of plant foods, which will dramatically reduce the total fat and saturated fat in your diet.
- Work up to one to two tablespoons of flaxseed oil each day, taking it with a sulfur-containing form of protein, such as skim milk or low-fat cottage cheese. This will provide you with adequate life-sustaining EFAs.
- Stop eating margarine, shortening, mayonnaise, and commercial salad dressings, to avoid the dangerous saturated and polyunsaturated fats in those products.[22] Do not buy foods with the words *hydrogenated* or *partially hydrogenated* on the label.
- Do not eat more than 20 percent of the calories you consume as dietary fat. For example, if you eat 2,000 calories a day, only 400 calories should be from fat. If you can limit yourself to only 10 to 15 percent

fat, that will be even better for your overall health. Eating 1,500 calories a day, which is recommended for most women, will require you to limit your fat intake to 300 calories.[23] In fact, a fat intake of 150 to 200 calories would be preferable. One tablespoon of olive oil contains 120 calories. One tablespoon of mixed omega-3, omega-6, and omega-9 oils contains 135 calories.

- Buy all oils stored in glass, rather than plastic, to avoid contamination of the oil by toxic, carcinogenic PCB's.

Changing the way you eat depends on changing the way you cook. I do not believe that it is possible to convert the typical high-fat American diet to a healthy diet. Instead, leaving most American food behind and learning to prepare dishes from foreign cuisines can lead us to improving our health. Middle Eastern food, with only small quantities of meat, is generally healthy and delicious, as are Mediterranean and many Asian cuisines. Check out international cookbooks, familiarize yourself with the products in ethnic grocery stores, and ask foreign-born friends to teach you simple, healthy dishes from their cultures. Be sure to read all food labels carefully for the presence of dangerous fats in processed foods.

As you begin to re-educate yourself about dietary fats, try to give this new approach to fats a one-year trial. You are likely to feel significantly better, gaining energy, and losing weight. By then, you will probably not want to return to eating the dangerous fats that may have contributed to compromising your health in the first place.

8

Environmental Toxins in Food

The FDA [federal Food and Drug Administration] has failed in its stated purpose of protecting the public from harmful substances being added to the food supply. Millions of lives are at stake—including those of future generations.

Russell Blaylock, M.D.

We know that the accumulation of toxic chemicals in the body compromises the immune system. Many scientists today associate toxic chemicals with the current epidemic of immune system diseases.

John Robbins

Where do we stand as a nation relative to chemical residues in our food? How safe is our food supply? What do we know about the pesticides, herbicides, insecticides, fungicides, antibiotics, hormones, and taste enhancers added to most of the foods we buy at our supermarkets? Are these substances toxic and therefore dangerous? Is there any scientific evidence to suggest that we should avoid these chemicals when possible? Is it true that toxic overload from these food chemicals and other environmental sources may be a significant cause of autoimmune disease? Should those of us with immune system illnesses be any more concerned than the general healthy public about eating foods containing these chemical residues?

Once I decided to search for answers to these challenging questions, I expected to pack my camel train and set out to find the balanced view on agricultural chemicals. I had little inkling, however, that my safari through the food chemicals debate would be so arduous. The camels and I struggled over some of the most mountainous terrain we had encountered in our long journey toward health, our way often obstructed by huge boulders of conflicting interpretations of the scientific literature.

When we finally descended into a caravansary, in the form of university and state government libraries, where I hoped to find unbiased information, we seemed to be caught between warring camps. One outpost, representing the food chemicals industry and many farmers' organizations, swears that there is little danger to us from these chemicals. The other garrison, representing the environmental, alternative health, and a segment of the orthodox medical communities, believes that there is great potential danger from eating foods containing these chemical residues. The intensity of the views of both camps led me to realize one thing for certain—the issue of chemical contamination of our food supply is highly politicized in this country.

A wide variety of synthetic chemicals possessing pesticidal action have been used in agriculture in this country since the early 1940s. The major families of these chemicals include chlorinated hydrocarbons (or organochlorines), organophosphorous pesticides, carbamates, and a newer class known as the pyrethoids. The residues that researchers most often are finding today in our food, in decreasing order, are those of organochlorines, organophosphates, and carbamate pesticides. Other less commonly encountered pesticide residues include fungicides, herbicides, and fumigants.[1]

In the United States, our scientific and medical communities have been slow to respond to the potential of these chemicals for causing illness. More germane to those of us with lupus, concern about the health implications of widespread pesticide use and its suspected role in autoimmune disease is just beginning to appear in the scientific literature. Attempting to remain outside the politics of this complex issue, my personal search through the literature on agricultural chemicals has led me to disturbing information that is particularly relevant for lupus patients.

Besides the many studies suggesting that these agricultural chemicals are toxic and potentially cancer causing, there are also studies questioning whether they actually can disrupt the immune system. Indeed, some of these studies indicate that food chemicals may affect the very cellular structure of the immune system. In the international publication *Journal of Toxicology and Environmental Health,* the authors of an article published in 1996 on the use of pesticides state:

> Because of the wide use of pesticides for domestic and industrial purposes, the evaluation of their immunotoxic effects is of major concern for public health. The association between autoimmune diseases and pesticide exposure has been suggested. A potential risk for the immune system should [be considered], especially . . . in compromised patients [such as] children and the elderly. Epidemiological studies of diseases related to immunosuppression or autoimmunity—lupus erythematosus, rheumatoid arthritis—are warranted.[2]

Certainly the chronically ill are as vulnerable as children and our aged population.

Many of us are aware that residues of these agricultural chemicals are present virtually everywhere on our planet today—in our oceans, lakes, soil, and water supplies, and even at the north and south poles, far from where they are used. They are damaging the wildlife in places as diverse as Florida, the rivers of England, the Baltic, the Arctic, the Great Lakes, and Lake Baikal in Siberia. The damage to wildlife as well as lab animals has served as a warning about symptoms that are on the rise in the human population.[3]

These chemical residues are evident nearly everywhere in our food chain. Organochlorine residues are found in two main food classes: dairy products and meat, fish, and poultry. The remaining organochlorine residues are distributed among the other food classes; garden fruits and leafy vegetables contain half of them. The organophosphates are detected mainly in dairy products and potatoes.[4] Many experts agree that toxic chemical overload, derived from residues in food sources and the broader environment, is a substantial threat to health and well-being in our world. My most burning personal question has been whether there is any evidence that these chemicals can cause autoimmune disease? Although SLE is not acknowledged by the medical community to be caused by environmental contamination, two news reports about unusually large numbers of lupus cases in two geographic areas suggest that there could be a link between environmental contamination and autoimmune disease.

The first of these reports concerns a mysterious cluster of lupus cases that developed in the border town of Nogales, Mexico, in 1994. Newspaper journalists discovered a ranch on the Mexican side of the border that had been dumping pesticides into streams and burning manure contaminated with pesticides. The ranch owners claimed that they could not afford to build a proper disposal system for the chemicals. Health department officials in New Mexico were examining the situation to try to determine whether toxic chemicals were a causative factor behind the lupus cases in that episode.[5] They were unable to prove conclusively that the environmental toxins were causing lupus.

A more recent perplexing cluster of cases of lupus and scleroderma (another autoimmune disease) has been documented in South Boston. State Senator Stephen F. Lynch has asked the state government to investigate in the wake of the 1997 death of his cousin from South Boston. When Lynch began talking with people in the area, he suspected that there were an abnormal number of cases of these two illnesses in the neighborhood. "There seems to be something going on here," he said. "I'm not sure if it's environmental [but] it seems to cross ethnic lines." State officials have confirmed the unusually high number of these two autoimmune illnesses and are conducting a study to try to determine the cause. Lynch said there has been much speculation about possible environmental sources.[6] Although it is unlikely that the health department will find conclusive evidence of environmental contamination as a cause of autoimmune disease in this instance, it seems prudent for those of us with lupus, as well as the general public, to remain alert to the possibility.

From my research, I've learned that the dangers of toxic chemicals are very real. They may make us ill and, equally alarming, also may hinder us from recovering from disease. According to Dr. Andrew Weil, these environmental toxins can damage the DNA, which contains the information needed for spontaneous healing. Without viable cellular DNA, we have little chance of ever regaining our health.[7] Against the backdrop of this disturbing information, in early 1999, I was sitting at the Corner Cafe on the campus of Evergreen State College in Olympia, lunching on organic vegetarian Greek pizza and drinking organic herbal tea. This student-run eatery is the place, I recalled, where I first began thinking about eating organic food many years ago. As a student in the mid-1980s at this small liberal arts school, I attended classes with many people for whom eating organic food was singularly important. Conversation often swirled around pesticides, antibiotics, and other chemicals in the food, soil, and air. These chemicals, said our science professors, could make us sick. And we were reading the research that supported that view.

The scientific studies indicated that agricultural chemical residues might damage the liver, provoking a variety of symptoms, such as mental confusion, depression, abnormal nerve reflexes, headaches, and depression. There was also a growing body of data that suggested that exposure to pesticides and herbicides could cause cancer. One of the problems with the research was that most of the studies were being conducted on animals rather than humans. Whether humans would react to the chemicals in the same ways as animals was difficult to establish. Furthermore, the data at that time could not document whether humans might be able to tolerate low levels of these chemical residues without adverse health effects.

Some instructors at Evergreen were doing more than questioning whether chemicals in our food and environment were a good idea. They also encouraged the administration to set up an organic farming program, where students could learn chemical-free, sustainable agriculture. On a beautiful five acres carved out of a Douglas fir forest, students today learn the reasons for growing food organically. One reason is to avoid potentially dangerous chemicals; another is to grow more nutrient-rich produce.

An important component of organic farming is understanding which natural nutrients to add to the soil to create a rich environment for plant roots. Synthetic fertilizers primarily are constituted of nitrogen, phosphorus, and potash, inorganic, or non–carbon-bearing, compounds. Their benefit is that they are immediately water soluble and therefore directly absorbed by plants. One of the primary problems with synthetic fertilizers, however, is that they seep into subterranean riparian areas (areas on the banks of natural watercourses, such as rivers), causing excessive algae growth, which in turn depletes the oxygen supply for all marine life.

Organic fertilizers, on the other hand, build soil structure and fertility. They may be complex, carbon-bearing compounds, such as soybean meal, or inorganic compounds, such as rock phosphate. Organic fertilizers work slowly and do not compromise water quality. Instead of being directly absorbed by plants, they are utilized by soil microorganisms. When these microorganisms die and decay, the plants consume this organic source of nutrients. Using organic fertilizers, therefore, allows plants to consume a broader range of nutrients than synthetic fertilizers provide them.

Another successful approach used in organic farming is companion planting, where crops that have an affinity are planted near each other. This gardening technique helps control weed and insect populations, consequently increasing the health and yield of all the plants. Without using herbicides to kill weeds, organic farming can be a labor-intensive approach to raising food crops. Students of sustainable agriculture spend plenty of time on their hands and knees pulling weeds that vie for soil nutrients and water, coaxing the nutritious, edible plants toward harvest.

In the summer and fall, I often strolled with classmates through the lushness of the organic farm. The farm manager showed us huge mounds of compost cooking away as it decomposed. Compost, he explained, is a critical element for the soil in that it provides high numbers of microorganisms, which make micronutrients available to the plants. In turn, the plants provide us with many nutrients when we include them in our meals. Soil that is not enriched in this way may produce attractive plants, but they generally will not contain high levels of nutrients. Learning all this helped us enjoy the visual delight and perfumed aroma of rows of sweet peas, snapdragons, asters, marigolds, dahlias, and roses planted among the corn, potatoes, and green beans. In the huge greenhouse grew juicy, sweet tomatoes and hot chili peppers. The raspberries, prunes, and apples were old varieties still carrying intense flavors. All of this, we marveled, was possible without the use of a single chemical.

Meanwhile, in the larger society, the agrochemical industry continued to purvey its chemicals, touting their promise to raise production and improve the cosmetics of our food. Farmers across America listened. Since the 1950s, they had been hearing about these "wonder chemicals" that would kill pests and weeds, stimulate growth, improve flavor, and increase yield. Being good business people, they jumped at the opportunity to increase their profits. There is a darker side of this supposed boon to agriculture: As early as the late 1970s the government was accumulating test evidence that our food supply was chemically contaminated and that this contamination could be dangerous for us. "The possible health effects of chemical contamination of the nation's food includes systemic toxicity, mutations, cancer, birth defects, and reproductive disorders."[8]

The fact is that during nearly fifty years of pesticide use in this country there has been growing evidence of human toxic chemical contamination. As early as 1951, low concentrations of chlorinated pesticides were documented in human milk. Even though DDT was banned in 1973, largely owing to the publication of Rachel Carson's book *Silent Spring,* this pesticide continues to be found in human milk today, though at decreasing concentrations as time passes.[9] The pesticides lindane, hexachlorobenzene, and dieldrin also continue to be found at detectable levels in human milk samples. Whether these chemicals are affecting our infants and very young children adversely is the subject of heated debate. A number of studies have documented the sharp rise in cases of childhood leukemia in the past twenty years. A 1987 study funded by the University of Southern California found that children living in homes where household and garden pesticides were used had as much as a sevenfold greater chance of contracting childhood leukemia.[10]

Do we have definitive data proving that agricultural chemicals cause illness? The answer is no. But we do have studies that strongly indicate a connection. Because the Food and Drug Administration (FDA) does not allow experiments concerning the effects of toxic chemicals to be conducted on humans, American research in this field has been hampered. Some European countries do permit such research; therefore, we generally must go to the European research for human studies and to U.S. research for animal studies.

In my search for agricultural chemical effects on the immune system, I came across alarming test results. In a study conducted in 1988, mice exposed to the pesticide dieldrin showed signs of suppressed lymphocytes of the spleen. These data suggest that cell-mediated immunity may be affected adversely by pesticide exposure. There is more evidence of the immunotoxic effects of pesticides. Nearly 70 percent of the rats and mice given captan, another pesticide, experienced depressed antibody formation and reduced T- and B-cell counts in the spleen. Moreover, ingesting the pesticides lindane, malathion, and dichlorophos caused the antibody levels of rabbits to drop, limiting their resistance to infection.[11] There are several missing links in this research. We don't know whether the amounts of the chemicals given to animals under laboratory conditions replicate the low-dose amounts in the environment to which human beings are exposed. We also don't know whether human immune systems react to toxicity in the same way that animal immune systems react.

Mention must be made of one of the few studies done on humans. In eastern Missouri, of 154 people exposed to the herbicide TCDD and 155 unexposed people, those who were exposed had higher numbers of abnormal T-cell subsets. This finding suggests that TCDD exposure can adversely affect the T-cell component of the immune system.[12] Many if not all of us with SLE have abnormal T-cell counts. It seems possible, therefore, that chemical toxicity may be one factor in the pathogenesis of SLE.

Additionally, there is reason for those of us with nervous system involvement to be concerned about pesticides, herbicides, and insecticides. These chemicals are all derivatives of nerve gases used in World War II to attack the nervous system. They can be extremely dangerous to any living creature. According to the National Research Council, "Certain classes of pesticides, including organophosphates, carbamates, and organochlorines, are known to have neurotoxic effects, especially as a result of high-dose acute exposure. There is insufficient data to track low-dose neurodevelopmental effects."[13] A pressing question that emerges from all these studies concerns the effects of long-term, low-dose exposure on those of us who are already ill. Many of us who are concerned about this issue believe that long-term exposure to even very low doses of toxic chemicals can contribute to our illness.

I found only one study dealing with the effects on the human immune system of low-dose exposure to a toxic chemical. Adult women eighteen to seventy years of age were examined for immune health in 1985. They had been drinking groundwater that was found to be contaminated with the carbamate pesticide aldicarb.

> Results suggested an association between consumption of aldicarb and T-cell subset abnormalities, elevated response to *Candida* stimulation, increased number of T8 cells, and increased percentage of T8 to T4 cells. The T-cell analyses were repeated on three more occasions and gave reproducible results. However, there was no self-reported clinical evidence of adverse health effects in the study groups.[14]

The weakness of this study is that there appears to have been no long-term follow-up to determine whether the abnormal T-cell levels might have provoked later illness. We also do not know how long the women had been drinking contaminated water before they were tested.

In 1988, I became very ill with a mysterious and debilitating condition. One of my worst symptoms was that I seemed to be reacting to nearly all the food I ate. I was dizzy and nauseous during and after meals, foggy in my thinking, and weak an hour after a meal. We wondered whether chemicals in the food bought at the supermarket might have caused or contributed to these reactions. Two naturopaths we consulted agreed that I could be chemically sensitive. At the same time, to help relieve the grueling, tedious hours of my illness, Steve and I began searching for an activity close to home that would get us outdoors to enjoy nature again. The answer came one January morning as the sun streamed into our bedroom. Steve looked out the window and said, "We have this perfect southern exposure. You need food you can safely eat, and I need activity. Let's start organic gardening. You draw up the plans, and I'll do the work."

This was an intriguing idea, but a quick survey of our soil made us wonder whether we should give up before we started. Our prairie acre had been flattened by a glacier, leaving little topsoil. Instead, we had six inches of clay, full of gravel. Beneath that was hardpan—dense gravel impermeable to water—which Steve's shovel could barely penetrate. This was definitely not a congenial environment for most plants, we agreed. Although we knew that it wouldn't be easy, we decided to try to create an oasis there. In February Steve removed rocks for days; then a truck delivered soil for the four raised beds he built. In went the rich soil and then the organic fertilizers, such as rock phosphate, soybean meal, kelp meal, bonemeal, and dolomite lime. For the final phase of soil-building he added composted horse manure. Once the eight-foot-high fence was up to discourage deer, we were ready to plant.

We planted seeds for cold weather crops first, working the soil with our fingers. Later, seeds for green beans, squash, and tomatoes waited in neat rows, eager to germinate. Because our springs are generally cold in the northwest, Steve built low plastic tents, called *cloches,* the French word for "bell." Market gardeners in France in the late nineteenth century used glass covers shaped like bells over individual plants, trapping heat and creating miniature "greenhouse effects." We used much larger cloches over whole raised beds, to encourage our seeds to germinate. Voila! By late April we were eating lettuce, peas, and spinach from our own garden. These sweet, crunchy edibles convinced us that it was an extremely good idea to grow plants in rich organic matter and abstain from using synthetic chemicals.

During much of the planting, weeding, and harvesting, I was too ill to work, so I sat near the garden visiting with Steve and our friends who were helping with the gardening. During those pleasant hours in the sun, I began to think of the human body and mind as a garden that requires tending to thrive. Our bodies need weeding to cleanse them of unhealthy habits and thoughts. Just as in companion planting, we humans also thrive in the company of companions who are nurturing and trustworthy. Our bodies and minds occasionally need crop rotation in the form of fresh ideas, new images, and novel practices, in order to grow, blossom, and produce fruit. With a healthy body and mind, as with a healthy garden, we want to create enough balance so that we need to spend only a small portion of our time weeding, focusing instead on productive cultivation.

I began to think about how much my physical body was like a plant. We were creating a nontoxic environment that was balanced for the maximum health of each plant. Adding organic soil amendments provided the root systems of our plants with the mineral nutrients they required to flourish. Exposing the leaves to light for photosynthesis allowed the plants to grow abundantly. This garden environment helped me understand what I wanted for my own body and mind—a nontoxic environment full of nourishment and light for my soul. I hoped to move from imbalance, due to the illness, to a condition of equilibrium again. The ancient Greeks called this state of complete physical, mental, and spiritual health *homeostasis.*

My body, it seemed to me, was like a plant needing a gentler hand to cultivate it so that it could thrive. Just as we don't completely understand cellular health in humans, we also don't entirely comprehend how the nourishment of plants occurs on a cellular level. But we do know that if we trust the older, organic process, if we feed plants chemically unadulterated material, plants will thrive. Early in my illness I had decided to take this organic approach to healing. By trusting the health of my mind and body to the older, purer, simpler techniques used in naturopathy and TCM, I believed those "gentler hands" would help me return to a healthy state.

Over the years of my illness and recovery, our gardens have become a refuge for me both physically and spiritually. With its peace and tranquillity, a garden can provide a psychic connection to life-forms other than our own. Time slows down, allowing contemplation. The garden is not a linear concept but a circular orb, inviting one to enter at many points, sit or stretch out in myriad places. In this gentle setting, one becomes conscious of energy forms constantly changing. Life and death are omnipresent as plants bear fruit and die back. One becomes acutely aware of the need for insects to pollinate and earthworms to aerate. Here, when we are not cultivating, we can daydream, nap, sketch, write, meditate, paint, or simply listen to insects buzzing in the intense summer heat.

Our first organic garden harvest was the talk of our country road. One neighbor decided to build raised beds, too, and grow vegetables organically. Visitors dropped in, wanting to see our gardens and talk to us about organic growing. We laughingly said that if we could do this in our soil in the northwest climate, anybody could do it. Steve's newfound enthusiasm led him to attend a sustainable agriculture conference sponsored by the state extension service and Oregon Tilth, an organization that teaches people to grow food organically. He returned convinced that our food supply is contaminated with pesticide residues that are dangerous to our health, and he announced that he was dedicated to growing and eating organically forever. Friends of ours living on a tiny city lot dug up their front yard, put up plastic cloches, and started raising organic produce fifteen feet from the cars, people, and dogs traversing their street. Even my father, a decades-long devotee of diazanon, a toxic insecticide, began to rethink his position on garden and lawn chemicals.

CHEMICAL RESIDUES IN OUR FRESH PRODUCE

Serving our fresh produce at meals helped me begin to eat again without feeling extremely ill. Much of the dizziness and nausea dissipated, and I stopped experiencing so much stomach pain. Although we had no clinical proof, we had experiential evidence that strongly suggested that I had been reacting to chemicals in my nonorganic food. Today evidence is accumulating that many of these agricultural chemicals are so dangerous they should be banned. Many of us who are concerned about the contamination of our environment believe that Congress must rise above the intense lobbying by the agricultural chemicals industry and some farmers' organizations, and allow the Environmental Protection Agency to ban some of these chemicals and strictly regulate the use of others, to protect the general public. Meanwhile, as we wait for the government to act, how can we protect ourselves from chemical residues in our food? Let's take a look at some of these chemicals found on our fresh produce, the health problems they may cause, and the ways we can avoid or minimize their presence in our meals.

In the book *Pesticide Alert*, the authors list thirty-eight pesticides commonly found on our fruits and vegetables. Between 1982 and 1985, the FDA analyzed perishables for pesticide residues and found that 64 percent of imported produce contained residues, compared with 38 percent of domestic produce.[15] Most of the vegetables and fruits listed had three to five pesticide residues, at least one of which is considered by scientists to be "especially hazardous."[16]

More recent studies continue to document chemical contamination of our vegetables and fruits. In March 1999, Consumers Union, which publishes *Consumer Reports,* stated its findings of pesticide residue levels for twenty-seven food categories, based on U.S. Department of Agriculture data gathered between 1994 and 1997. They found seven foods—apples, grapes, green beans, peaches, pears, spinach, and winter squash—with toxicity scores up to hundreds of times higher than the other foods tested. One reason is that farmers generally use more pesticides on these crops. Apples, for example, contained thirty-seven different chemicals, compared with broccoli with ten chemicals. A second reason is that fruits and vegetables with a high pesticide residue are treated with more toxic pesticides and often eaten unpeeled. Other produce, including sweet corn, frozen or canned peas, orange juice, milk, canned peaches, bananas, broccoli, and apple juice, had lower scores.[17]

Consumers Union takes a conservative position by stating that a "high toxicity score doesn't automatically mean that a food is unsafe to eat."

Our risk, they say, depends on our age, our susceptibility to the specific pesticide compound, the number of times we eat the particular food, and the amount we eat relative to our body size. While this advice may be appropriate for the healthy public, I believe that it is too conservative an approach for children and those of us who are already ill. Children are at the most risk, because they eat far more produce per pound of body weight than adults and they are more sensitive to some effects of pesticides. As lupus patients, we need to reduce the chemical load in our bodies as much as possible. Even extremely low residue levels of many of these compounds can affect the nervous system. Some of these compounds may interfere with endocrine gland functions, and the research supports the possibility that these chemicals cause cancer.

The weakness inherent in the Consumers Union analysis is that they ignore most of the chemicals being used on our food and discuss only three pesticides that they say are the worst: methylparathion, dieldrin, and aldicarb. Keeping in mind that these three chemicals are only the tip of the iceberg, a brief discussion of each may help us understand the enormity of the problem we are facing.

Methylparathion is an organophosphate, which means that it has been designed to attack insects by poisoning their neurologic systems. Organophosphates work the same way in humans as in insects. Is methylparathion dangerous to us? After all, we are huge creatures compared with insects. The answer lies in a statement made by the Environmental Protection Agency (EPA) in 1998 that concluded that methylparathion creates an "unacceptable risk" at the levels allowed at present. National agriculture statistics show that U.S. farmers are using less of this insecticide on peaches than in 1996 but more on apples and green beans.

The most toxic of all pesticides is aldicarb. Not only does it cover the outside of the produce but it also permeates the flesh of the vegetable and so cannot be washed off. Most growers stopped using it in 1990, but some potato growers in Washington and Idaho stepped up its use again in the late 1990s.

The third-worst chemical, according to Consumers Union, is dieldrin. A carcinogenic (meaning "cancer-causing") pesticide, dieldrin was taken off the market in 1974, but it carries as much risk as other chemicals still in use, because it takes decades to disappear from the soil. Dieldrin also is absorbed into the pulp of vegetables. Root crops, such as potatoes, and vine crops, such as cucumbers, squash, and melons, are particularly susceptible to absorbing dieldrin. This chemical poses a definite health risk. A study published in 1976 in Denmark found that women with higher levels of the pesticide dieldrin in their blood had a greater risk of breast cancer.[18]

Is anything being done to protect us from these dangerous agricultural chemicals? After the National Academy of Sciences issued a report on pesticides in children's diets, Congress responded with the Food Quality Protection Act passed unanimously in 1996. This act empowers the EPA to regulate pesticide use. The weakness of this new legislation, in the minds of many of us concerned about food issues, is that it allows the EPA to establish risk-tolerance levels. Many of us wonder how the EPA will know where to set the tolerance levels when there do not appear to have been adequate studies leading to valid conclusions about the risks these chemicals pose for humans.

Still, the EPA is beginning to make some headway. It has lowered the "safe" limit for nineteen of forty organophosphate pesticides. In August 1999 the agency debated whether to further restrict or ban certain pesticides, including all organophosphates. As of January 2000 the pesticides methylparathion and azinphos-methyl have been banned. As you might guess, the banning of these chemicals is undergoing intense debate in Congress. Agricultural chemical companies and some farmers are arguing that the government should not overly restrict pesticides. The fact is, though, as I pointed out earlier in this chapter, there are organic ways of controlling pests and weeds that do not require the use of synthetic chemicals at all. But the agri-chemical producers continue to push for use of their toxic pesticides on our food.

As lupus patients, we need to avoid food that contains chemical residues. The challenges of accomplishing this may seem too difficult at first, but the good news is that there are a number of ways you can protect yourself from these toxins. Ideally, all fresh produce should be labeled to identify where the food was grown and what pesticide residues it contains, thus allowing consumers to make informed choices. This consumer protection legislation does not yet exist, but many of us are hoping that it will be implemented in the near future. Meanwhile, we must inform ourselves and be vigilant in the produce section of the grocery store.

At the very least, we should not eat supermarket produce with the highest toxicity scores. These include peaches, winter squash, green beans, pears, spinach, apples, and grapes. We should be sure to peel all supermarket produce or wash it with dilute dishwashing detergent in a sink full of water. To remove pesticide residue from green beans, leafy vegetables, grapes, and strawberries, swirl them in a dilute (one teaspoon dish detergent per gallon of water at room temperature) solution for five to ten seconds, and then rinse in slightly warm water. For firmer vegetables and fruits, use a soft brush to scrub the food with the same solution and rinse in warm water. A study conducted by the Southwest Research Institute in San Antonio, Texas, showed that this method eliminated or substantially reduced pesticide residues on seventeen popular fruits and vegetables.[19] It's important to remember, however, that while washing and scrubbing will remove surface sprays, it will not eliminate the systemic chemicals, such as aldicarb, that may be in the pulp itself as a result of absorption through the roots.

Another way to cut back on your exposure to these toxic chemicals is to can or freeze fruits and vegetables. A study conducted by the National Food Processors Association states that washing and blanching produce for freezing or canning eliminates nearly all pesticide residue. The lead scientist in that study found that 83 percent of residues of the commonly used fungicide benomyl, which scientists suspect causes birth defects, was removed when apples were made into applesauce.[20] This may be biased information (this organization represents the food industry), but there is agreement from a nonindustry source. The nonprofit Environmental Working Group states, "Canned fruits and vegetables usually contain much lower levels of pesticide residues than fresh."[21]

The best way to avoid chemical contamination is to buy organic produce, which has little or no pesticide residues. How can we be sure the "organic" food we buy is really organic? We need tough regulations and on-site inspections. At present, the state of Washington has one of the most stringent programs in the country for certifying organic produce. In this state, certified organic farms are inspected at least once a year to ensure two things: first, that there have been no applications of synthetic fertilizers or synthetic pesticides for at least three years before harvest, and second, that the farmer is using a soil-building program that provides for healthy soil and healthy plants. Organic pest control relies on crop rotation and the possible use of nontoxic insecticidal soaps, dormant oils, or botanical insecticides, such as neem or pyrethrum. All materials used in organic food production are required to be derived from a natural source and not harmful to human health or the environment when used appropriately.[22]

In Washington there are more than five hundred growers, processors, and handlers of organic food bringing in more than $60 million in sales each year. Your state also may have a healthy organic food industry. Call your state's Department of Agriculture and ask for information on their certified organic farming program. If the state doesn't have one, contact your legislators, requesting that such a program be started. One of the ways we can clean up our food is to become food activists.

Although organic food is more expensive than nonorganic food, we have noticed in the past three years that prices are dropping significantly compared with those we paid ten years ago. Often, the price for organic lettuce at our local food cooperative is the same or slightly lower than nonorganic supermarket lettuce. To soften the impact of organic food on our budget, we use a shopping guideline: If the organic item is up to 50 percent more expensive than the nonorganic item, we buy it. If it is more costly, we don't purchase it. If you are unable to find organic produce at your supermarket, request that the management start carrying it. The more requests they have, the higher the likelihood that they will begin stocking it. Read labels carefully to be certain that produce is certified organic according to state agriculture department requirements.

Another excellent way to find organic food is to join a local food cooperative. We have belonged to ours for nearly twenty years. We pay a yearly membership fee, which in turn pays salaries to the managers. Stockers and cashiers volunteer their time in return for a discount on their food purchases. Our food co-op provides a children's play area inside and an outdoor free clothing bin. Co-op membership gives us access to certified organic fruit and vegetables from California during the winter. Knowing we are eating safe food brings us great peace of mind.

Get a group together, pool your money, and arrange to purchase in bulk from an organic foods wholesaler. If you are too ill to organize the project, ask a friend or family member to help. You can distribute the food to your members from your garage or porch. Eventually, your membership may grow to a point where you can rent a small storefront or warehouse and hire an employee or two. During the summer we grow much of our own organic produce. We also are experimenting with winter gardening of mixed salad greens grown under cloches, which worked last winter until freezing temperatures arrived. Do join a local food co-op if you can find one. If you can't, why not start one?

If you are unable to grow some of your own food because of lack of space or the difficult symptoms of your illness, you may be able to find a farm in your area that is involved in a Community Supported Agriculture (CSA) program. This movement began in Europe about twenty-five years ago. Today there are more than six hundred CSA farms in the United States. For a fee, members buy a share of the food crops. During the growing season, boxes of fresh, organic produce arrive at your front door every week. Some CSAs even allow you to work off part of your monthly fee by helping with the weeding and harvesting. During the two years we belonged to a CSA, we received not only big boxes of delicious vegetables and fruit, but also old-fashioned flower bouquets. Also enclosed were invitations to attend picnics and hayrides at the farm, where we were able to buy from larger crops—such as potatoes, tomatoes, basil, and corn—at lower-than-retail prices.

This is an excellent way to participate in farming without having to own and run a farm. It's also a way to support small, family-owned farms, which are the primary providers of organic produce to those of us who are intent upon eating clean food. Contact your state's Department of Agriculture for a list of CSA farms in your region, or use the contact information in the resource section of this book. If there are no CSAs near you, look for an organic farmer who understands the concept and work with him or her to get a membership farm started. Talk up the idea with your friends and offer to bring the farmer an initial group of members to help the CSA get off the ground.

If you cannot garden for financial reasons, you might be able to find a Kitchen Garden Project in your area that would help you set up your gardens for free. These dedicated volunteers will come to your home or apartment, set up the raised beds, fill them with good soil, and provide you with plant seeds. They also will teach you how to plant, weed, water, and harvest. This service is helping many low-income people in our county eat nontoxic, fresh produce.

If you can't afford to buy organically or you can't find a source of organic food in your area, you may decide to take the risk of eating the least contaminated supermarket produce. This includes United States-grown tomatoes, carrots, and broccoli as well as oranges, wheat, sweet potatoes, canned or frozen peas, bananas, orange juice, milk, and canned or frozen corn.[23] If you eat this same food imported from other countries, it may contain much higher pesticide residues. Remember that there are chemical residues on nearly all supermarket produce unless it is certified organic. While fresh produce from Mexico is being found to be less contaminated with chemicals than is produce grown in this country, that does not mean Mexican produce is safe. The only way to protect yourself and your family from these dangerous chemicals is to eat organically.

CHEMICALS IN PROCESSED FOODS

Thus far, we have talked only about chemical contamination of fresh produce. But processed, packaged foods also contain chemicals that can affect our health adversely. Although animal test results suggest that some of these additives cause cancer, the FDA so far has concluded that they don't pose a significant cancer risk to humans. Like agricultural chemicals, the arena of processed food chemical additives is also highly political. For example, the FDA recommended that red dye no. 3 be banned, based on evidence that it caused thyroid tumors in rats. That recommendation was overruled by pressure from the Reagan Administration. Since those of us with lupus are in a weakened physical state, we may be more susceptible to adverse effects from the worst of these food additives. A brief discussion of the most suspicious additives and where they're found can help us decide which packaged foods to avoid.

There are a number of food additives and food coloring agents that are potentially harmful. The first is **acesulfame K,** which is found in chewing gum, diet soft drinks, frozen desserts, gelatin products, no-sugar-added baked goods, and Sunett, a tabletop sweetener recently approved by the FDA for addition to soft drinks. Poorly designed studies conducted in the 1970s suggest that this food additive causes cancer.

Another food additive to avoid is **aspartame,** also called Nutrasweet, which contains aspartate. Aspartame is found in such diet foods as drink mixes, frozen desserts, no-sugar-added gelatin, soft drinks, and the table-top sweetener called Equal. Some tests indicate that it causes cancer. Furthermore, the FDA has received many complaints that it produces allergic reactions. More important, evidence now exists that aspartate affects the nervous system and spinal cord, promoting brain neurons to die, and thus leading to neurologic diseases, such as Parkinson's, Alzheimer's, and Lou Gehrig's disease (amyotrophic lateral sclerosis). It also damages the brains of infants and children, who then have a higher that normal propensity for suffering neurologic diseases later in their lives.[24] Aspartate also has been shown to produce tumors in animal testing.[25]

One of the worst of these food additives is the new fat substitute called **olestra,** sold under the brand name Olean. This is a synthetic fat that can cause severe diarrhea, loose stools, abdominal cramps, and intestinal gas. It also limits the body's ability to absorb carotenoids, such as beta-carotenes, from fruits and vegetables. Carotenoids are precisely the compounds that may lower our risk of cancer and heart disease. I have had a severe reaction to this additive; my medical doctor suspects that it is present in a low-fat cracker I ate. Since the FDA does not require that olestra be included on ingredient labels, my doctor is warning her patients to stay away from low-fat products.

Other food additives to avoid include saccharin, sodium nitrate and sodium nitrite and potassium bromate. **Saccharin,** an additive which has been around for years, can cause cancer of the uterus, ovaries, skin, blood vessels, and other organs, according to numerous animal studies. **Sodium nitrate** and **sodium nitrite** are used in bacon, corned beef, frankfurters, ham, luncheon meat, and smoked fish. According to studies, they introduce only a small cancer risk, but it's worth avoiding them. **Potassium bromate,** a flour enhancer, is used to increase the volume of bread. Banned in the United Kingdom in 1989 because of its cancer-causing effects in animals, it rarely is used in the United States and particularly not in California, because state law there requires that any product including it carry a cancer warning.

An extremely toxic food chemical is **monosodium glutamate** (MSG). As a taste enhancer, it is found in many packaged and processed foods, such as chips, frozen entrées, restaurant food, salad dressing, and packaged soups. The least difficulty with this chemical is that it can cause headaches. In children, it provokes endocrine disorders, learning disabilities, autism, dyslexia, and emotional control disorders, such as violent behavior and paranoia.[26] MSG also is strongly suspected to be a leading stimulus to neurodegenerative diseases that adults suffer late in their lives from the cumulative effects of eating it over many years. An animal study published in 1991 is of special interest to those of us with lupus. In this study baby mice exposed to MSG were found to have a severe defect in cell-mediated immunity when they reached adulthood.[27] **Cysteine** and **hydrolyzed vegetable protein** are also taste enhancers used throughout the packaged food industry; these two additives also can cause neurologic damage, because they contain 20 percent to 60 percent MSG as well as aspartate.

Most artificial colorings in foods are of little nutritional value. While we all would benefit from further testing, animal tests to date suggest an association with various forms of cancer. The ones to avoid as much as possible are: **blue dye no. 1,** in baked goods, beverages, and candy; **blue dye no. 2,** in beverages, candy, and pet food; **green dye no. 3**, in beverages and candy; **red dye no. 3**, in baked goods, candy, and cherries in fruit cocktail; **red dye no. 40**, in candy, gelatin desserts, pastries, and pet food; and **yellow dye no. 6**, in baked goods, beverages, candy, gelatin, and sausage.[28] Because chemicals are present in so much of our processed, packaged food, the best approach for those of us who are ill is to eat as little packaged food as possible.

CHEMICALS IN MEAT AND DAIRY PRODUCTS

Thus far, we have dealt with chemicals in fresh produce and packaged foods. What about our meat, dairy, and fish supplies? Are these food sources cleaner and therefore safer to eat? In a word, no. The fact is that many of our animal protein foods are contaminated with antibiotics, hormones, and fungicides as well as pesticide residues derived from animal feed. A 1994 report by the EPA found that meats and cheeses are a major source of dioxin exposure in the United States today.[29]

We have known about pesticide-, fungicide-, antibiotic-, and hormone-contaminated meat, fish, and dairy for more than twenty-five years. As early as 1976, the FDA published test results that estimated that 1.9 million tons of beef and 1.1 million tons of swine with residues of pesticides and animal drugs were sold to the public that year alone.[30] This was the era of the Delaney Clause, when any agricultural chemical residues were illegal. Today the use of pesticides, antibiotics, hormones, and fungicides in the raising of our feed animals is entirely legal under guidelines established by the government. Even though ranchers and factory farmers use huge amounts of these chemicals, many scientific researchers and health professionals persist in warning that they are dangerous to the public health. As with the controversy surrounding chemical contamination of fresh produce, the animal drug and farming industries claim there are insufficient studies on humans to document adverse health effects of these chemical residues in meat, milk, and eggs. That does not mean, however, that these chemicals are safe. As Dr. Jere Goyan, past commissioner of the FDA, has said, "When it comes to using drugs and chemicals in meat animals, we find ourselves in a situation in which our problems are well ahead of our answers."[31]

To better comprehend this situation, let's first take a look at the risk of antibiotic residues in our meat supply. The problem stems from the fact that antibiotics in animal feed create transferable drug resistance—livestock bacteria that becomes resistant to antibiotics can eventually lead to drug resistance in human bacteria as a result of our consumption of this antibiotic-laced meat. Doctors began realizing as early as 1955 that people were contracting dysentery caused by a pathogen resistant to all the antibiotics targeted to treat it. They began to suspect that the origins of this problem went back to the late 1940s when many new antibiotics were created—penicillin, streptomycin, chloramphenicol, tetracycline, and chlortetracycline. Sensing a great business opportunity, pharmaceutical firms began manufacturing antibiotics for animal feed-additive use. By 1954 our livestock—cattle, hogs, and chickens—were being fed antibiotics; by 1984, the amount of antibiotics used reached nearly nine million pounds.[32]

Interestingly, as of 1984, ranchers using subtherapeutic doses of antibiotics still didn't really know what these drugs accomplished. They theorized that antibiotics might make the animals grow faster by limiting subclinical disease. The farmers did know for certain that these drugs increased the weight of their animals, which raised their profits. Now scientists believe that, over time, the antibiotics tampering with the DNA structure of pathogens found in these animals is creating strains of bacteria that are completely resistant to all the antibiotics used in treating human illnesses. Such organizations as the American Pork Congress and National Cattlemen's Association continue to lobby Congress to be allowed to use these drugs. According to many doctors, these antibiotics are prompting a quiet public health crisis that is only just beginning to be reported in the national press.

As lupus patients, we need to be particularly alert to this problem. We often are prone to infections and count on the effectiveness of antibiotics to help our already overburdened immune systems cope with killing infectious agents. Now that there are so many pathogens that are resistant to antibiotics, we are at risk of not being able to find drugs that will kill our infections. I have a low-grade stomach infection that has proved resistant to all the antibiotics my doctors have prescribed to kill it. This pathogen clearly has had a chance to adapt to antibiotics.

Another potential problem for people who eat meat is the injection of hormones into meat animals. The synthetic estrogen diethylstilbestrol, or DES, was detected in beef in the 1960s. Used as a growth promoter in meat animals from the 1950s, DES also was given in the 1960s and 1970s to pregnant women to prevent miscarriages. In 1971, the *New England Journal of Medicine* published findings that a form of cancer of the vagina called clear-cell adenocarcinoma was developing in many daughters born to these women.[33] DES also was found to be generating symptoms of impotence, infertility, enlarged breasts, or changes in the voice register among farmers who inhaled DES in powdered form. DES finally was banned in 1979 over strong objections from the animal drug industry, but the ban did not stop its use. In the spring of 1980, a scandal erupted when the FDA found this illegal hormone still implanted in 427,275 head of cattle in 318 different feedlots in twenty states.[34] There is growing evidence that DES-exposed women have a greater likelihood of experiencing autoimmune diseases, such as Graves' disease, rheumatoid arthritis, and other diseases stemming from defects in the regulation of the immune system.[35]

Today there is a lucrative market for growth-promoting hormones, and large drug companies are promoting these products aggressively to feedlot producers. One popular hormonal feed additive contains the estrogen estradiol; another contains synthetic progesterone. Yet another is a combination of estradiol, testosterone, and progesterone. Feedlots also use hormones as tranquilizers. The scientific community has run many studies that show that these hormones are potentially carcinogenic.

For lupus patients, a warning about hormone residues in our food supply is important. Some lupus researchers suspect that female hormones cause or perpetuate lupus. A 1998 study reported in the *British Journal of Rheumatology* states that "there is ample evidence that female sex hormones affect the incidence and disease course of SLE."[36] Sex hormones are found throughout our meat and milk supply. Pork and chicken tested in Philadelphia in the early 1980s showed high levels of hormone residues.

Milk samples taken at the same time revealed low levels of estrogens.[37] Any hormone residue, in my opinion, could be significant for lupus patients.

Milk cartons have been found by FDA testing to be a significant source of dioxin, an organochlorine. Dioxin is present in the chlorine-bleaching process of the paper used to make the cartons. This is relevant for lupus patients, because dioxin is known to cause immune system depression, specifically by damaging the thymus gland.[38] It also can produce birth defects, behavioral and learning problems, miscarriage, lowered sperm count, liver disease, and genetic damage. All of us who drink milk from bleached cartons are being exposed to low-level dioxin.

Is this exposure to dioxin necessary? Definitely not. As an expert witness stated when appearing before a U.S. House of Representatives hearing in 1989:

> The question we should be debating today is not how much dioxin is too much, but why we should be forced to ingest dioxin at all. It is very simple to produce a dioxin-free milk carton. You simply don't bleach it. These are in use in countries like Sweden and Australia where governments and companies cite environmental concern in their decision to produce these cheaper products.[39]

As of 1999, the EPA had not required the pulp and paper industry to adopt technology that would limit the dioxin and other toxic pollutant content of their products. In 1998 the National Wildlife Federation instituted a lawsuit, which is still pending, against the EPA for failing to ban dioxin. The lawsuit is demanding that the EPA tighten recently issued regulations for the pulp and paper industry. The federation wants the EPA to require technology that will move the industry closer to the eventual adoption of a totally chlorine-free paper process. Now in use in Europe, this process produces no chlorine, significantly reduces other pollutants, and uses one eighth of the energy required by chlorine-based processes.[40] Some U.S. paper companies have begun to substitute nonchlorine bleaches, such as oxygen and hydrogen peroxide, which release no dioxins, but until the EPA establishes a complete ban on dioxin, consumers trying to protect their health would be wise to avoid products that contain dioxin residues. These include bleached milk cartons, coffee filters, paper diapers, paper plates, tea bags, storage cartons, and women's sanitary products.

There are additional agricultural chemicals in use around cattle, sheep, pigs, and chickens. In the crowded and unsanitary conditions in which they are raised, cattle and sheep are doused with toxaphene, a chlorinated hydrocarbon, to kill the parasites that breed in these crowded conditions. Toxaphene is therefore considered one of the most toxic and deadly insecticides. There are documented cases of death of many feedlot animals exposed to this pesticide.[41] Toxaphene has seeped into our water supply from food crops and factory farm use, and it has contaminated our broader environment, killing wildlife, particularly birds, at high rates. It also has been found to be contaminating fish.[42] Even worse, toxaphene has been proved to cause cancer. Dr. Melvin Reuber, a pathologist and toxicology specialist who served as a research scientist for the National Cancer Institute and as a consultant to the EPA, stated that the results of a thirty-year study of toxaphene left no doubt that "toxaphene is such a carcinogen it boggles the mind."[43]

Chemical contamination of our fish supply is also evident. PCBs, which are chlorinated hydrocarbons, have contaminated many of the planet's lakes and oceans. Fish have been absorbing extremely high concentrations of toxaphene and other chemicals from their watery environments for decades. Shellfish also accumulate high concentrations of pesticides, and humans take in PCBs by eating contaminated fish and shellfish. Because our livestock and chickens are fed huge quantities of fish meal, they, too, have become contaminated with the toxic residues present in fish.

Chicken is a source of animal protein that many of us particularly enjoy. Is there a chance that the chickens we buy at the supermarket are any freer of residues than other meats? Virtually none. The story of chicken factory farming in the United States is not pretty. These chickens are fed a steady diet of sulfa drugs, hormones, antibiotics, and nitrofurans as well as arsenic compounds.[44] The birds' diets are very poor nutritionally. Broilers' food is regulated strictly to maximize their weight. Layers' diets are created only to boost egg production. As a result of severe vitamin deficiencies, these chickens often are diseased, suffering such ailments as blindness, bone and muscle weakness, brain damage, and internal bleeding. Chickens at these farms often are kept crushed together in tiny cages, unable to lift a wing or even turn around. They also are kept away from natural sunlight. A major problem many of us face in eating these chickens is the chemical residues in their flesh. Equally disturbing, however, is the cruel treatment of these highly social creatures.

Once I realized that I should not be eating commercial chicken because of the antibiotic and hormone residues, we went in search of chemical-free, affordable chicken. One evening I brought up the subject in our voluntary simplicity study circle. Was anyone else interested in eating organic, humanely raised chicken? "Yes," said some members of the group. We contacted the new owners of a forty-acre farm, who were returning their land to an organic, sustainable model after years of neglect as a dairy farm. Would they, we asked, be willing to grow organic chickens for us if we brought them customers? They were enthusiastic about the idea, since they had been studying *Pastured Poultry Profits,* which explains how to raise chickens organically and humanely for profit.[45]

The first summer, these farmers raised two cycles of chickens, sixty-five in each round, housed in a cleverly designed pen that they moved each day through one of their pastures. Because chickens are prone to many diseases, instead of giving them antibiotics, the owners had each chick vaccinated at a small cost. The chicks thrived in the open air, able to scratch and peck at the ground while they ate only state-certified organic feed. As the farmers moved the pens each day, the chicken droppings spread lightly to eliminate pollution and encourage lush, green grass for young lambs to graze on in the summer.

Each summer the project repeats, with healthy chickens living in fresh air, sunshine, and clean pasture. In addition to their organic feed, they eat grass and insects to supplement their diets. The farmers comment happily that this is true sustainable agriculture, in which most farming activities are interdependent and few, if any, chemicals are used. In the five years of production there has been only one small outbreak of disease.

The birds are presold each spring to bring the farmers enough cash to purchase and feed the chickens. The customer pays the balance of the price per pound when they pick up the butchered chickens in July. We purchase twenty-five organic chickens per year, freeze them, and serve them twice a month. They are more flavorful than factory-raised chickens, with that "Grandma's chicken and dumpling" taste. They are also much less fatty than commercially raised chickens and are completely free of antibiotics and hormones. Very important to many of us is the peace of mind of knowing that the chickens are humanely cared for while they are alive.

Lupus patients would be well advised to avoid nonorganic chicken. If you are unable to find certified organic chicken, consider starting a small backyard flock of your own. Or perhaps you can find a farmer near you who would like to be involved in this profitable venture. You also can keep laying hens, feeding them organically to ensure a good supply of organic eggs. Chickens need to be properly housed to protect them from bad weather and predators, such as cats, rats, raccoons, and weasels. Chicks and chickens also need enough room to walk and socialize in their flock as well as a relatively quiet environment to lay plenty of eggs.

I cannot stress strongly enough that as a lupus patient you should stop eating commercially raised beef, lamb, pork, and chicken. Determine to find organically raised meat. If that is not possible, move to eating soy products for protein that is made from organic soy and combinations of organic brown rice and organic beans, also a protein source. There are reasons to eat organic food beyond avoiding the danger of chemical residue. Food that is grown organically is generally of high nutritive value and more flavorful than non-organic food, particularly if you purchase it fresh. Organic farming methods encourage biodiversity by building soil nutrients and rotating crops. Another benefit of organic farming is that it protects the water supply not only by conserving water but also by avoiding chemical wastes that contaminate water. By eating organically, we also contribute to the health of farmworkers. Illnesses triggered by agricultural chemicals among farmworkers are occurring at alarming rates. Workers on organic farms are safer from the likelihood of contracting occupationally related disease.

Until recently, most regulation of organic standards has been done on a state-by-state basis. In 1999, the U.S. Department of Agriculture finally announced that it would allow the term *organic* to be used on meat and poultry, meaning that it has been raised without the use of antibiotics and synthetic hormones, fed only organic feed, and processed in accordance with accepted organic standards. Packaged foods also will be eligible for the organic label if 95 percent of the ingredients are organic. Dairy products can carry the organic label, too, if milk cows are certified as not fed antibiotics or synthetic hormones and their milk is processed according to organic standards.

One important cautionary note: Be careful about food labels that state "pesticide free," or "grown without chemical fertilizers." These are useless terms that do not in any way mean the product is organic. The only way to be sure that you are eating organic food is to buy foods labeled "certified organic." Those words assure you that the conditions in which your food is grown and processed are being inspected by an objective organization that, by law, can certify that the food you buy is organic.

9

The Dangers of Toxic Dentistry

The Academy has serious concerns regarding the American Dental Association's lack of scientific rigor and the tendency to misinform the dental profession and, thereby, the public at large regarding the established facts about (mercury) amalgam safety. . . . This failure has resulted in inadequate protection to the public . . . from personal harm due to amalgam usage.

International Academy of Oral Medicine and Toxicology[1]

Have you ever wondered whether your lupus could be connected to your dental fillings? Although I certainly had never thought of that, I began to suspect that there was something very wrong in my mouth when I showed signs of periodontal disease some months into my mystery illness. Even though I had taken diligent care of my teeth since childhood, I had many fillings. Once the illness set in, my gums became swollen and tender to the touch and bled when I brushed my teeth. Because I was so ill, I felt that I could not endure dental procedures at that time. I had to wait many months until I was strong enough to walk up the flight of stairs to my dentist's office. The results of his examination were disappointing but not surprising. He told me that two molars would have to be pulled and that I would need scraping under the gum line and a medicated mouthwash to control the gingivitis.

I suspected that there were more problems in my mouth than just those molars and periodontal disease, however. Thinking back over my illness, I recalled that I first began to experience fatigue, vertigo, heart palpitations, eczema, and vision problems after I had undergone a root canal procedure and had a crown placed in my mouth in the late 1970s. Within three months of that procedure I could not make it through a tennis match. Within less than a year, a goiter developed, and a hyperactive thyroid gland was diagnosed. My doctor at the time told me that this was an autoimmune disease. He was mystified as to why I was experiencing the problem, since there was no history of goiter in my family and I had eaten seafood regularly—a source of the iodine necessary for a healthy thyroid gland.

My doctor's attempts to curb the hyperactivity of my thyroid without an invasive procedure failed, and I was left with the difficult choice of having my thyroid gland surgically removed or deactivated by radioactive iodine. I chose the radioactive iodine. After that treatment, I became very ill as my level of thyroid hormone dropped sharply. Then I was prescribed a synthetic thyroid hormone, which I would have to take for the rest of my life, because I had no thyroid function left.

Ten years later, when I became ill with my mystery illness, I wondered whether the source might be in my teeth. Loading my camel caravan again to search for healing, I was unaware that this would be the most difficult of all my safaris. I was soon to learn that the rhetoric surrounding the mercury amalgam issue was so shrill that it seemed nearly impossible to find clear scientific data that would offer a balanced view of the issue. As my camels and I struggled through the ferocious sandstorms swirling around us, I nearly gave up and called off the quest. But the image of the Karamojong warriors came back to me, signaling me to be courageous and alert. Then my husband found two books on mercury dental amalgams that persuaded me to continue the journey: *It's All in Your Head*, by Hal Huggins, and *Mercury Poisoning from Dental Amalgam: A Hazard to Human Brain*, by Patrick Stortebecker. As I read Dr. Huggins's collection of anecdotal accounts about the dangers of mercury amalgam fillings, I recognized many of my own symptoms. Reading Dr. Stortebecker's scientific account of the dangers of mercury amalgam was even more alarming, since it documented the possible brain and nervous system damage from mercury exposure. I wondered whether I could have low-level mercury poisoning from my dental amalgams. Might that be causing my illness? Of the thirty-four possible symptoms of "amalgam syndrome" listed in Huggins' book, I was experiencing seventeen: eczema, thyroid malfunction, gastrointestinal irritation, depression, weakness of muscles, bleeding gums, a sour and metallic taste in my mouth, balance problems, hearing problems, vertigo, impaired capacity to do intellectual work, difficulty making decisions, dry eyes, irregular heartbeat, fatigue, anxiety, and vision problems.[2]

I also was startled to learn that mercury in dental amalgams is not the only potential hazard of modern dentistry. According to Dr. Huggins, the electrical current created by the various metals that make up "silver" dental fillings can interfere with brain waves, causing neurologic problems. I knew that I had twenty-two amalgam fillings, one root canal filling, and two crowns that were part metal and part porcelain. That added up to a mouth full of metal that, in light of this new information, could be compromising my health. We were alarmed by all of this information, and quickly located other scientific sources on mercury dental amalgams, to broaden our knowledge of the subject.

The story that unfolded was shocking. Mercury is the most toxic nonradioactive element on earth. At the worst, exposure to mercury can cause people to go mad, become severely physically debilitated, and die. The Hatter, a character in Lewis Carroll's *Alice's Adventures in Wonderland*, is mad as a result of occupational exposure to mercury, used during the nineteenth century in the felt-curing process involved in making the top hats that were in style during that era. Doctors and scientists at that time *knew* that mercury was the source of the madness of those in the hatter's trade.

The Chinese were using small amounts of mercury mixed with other metals to plug cavities in the teeth as early as the seventh century. They probably picked mercury because it is easier to work with than other metals and does not deteriorate. Throughout the Middle Ages, alchemists in China and Europe observed that this mysterious silvery liquid, extracted from cinnabar ore, was volatile and would disappear quickly as vapor when mildly heated. Although they were aware of the dangers of mercury, early-nineteenth-century French dentists nevertheless began mixing mercury with various other metals to fill cavities in teeth. These early mixtures had little mercury in them, but by 1833, when amalgams were introduced to the United States, they contained significantly more mercury. This alarmed many scientists and dentists. In fact, opposition was so strong to mercury amalgams that the American Society of Dental Surgeons required its members to sign pledges promising not to use mercury amalgams. In 1848, the society found eleven of its New York members guilty of malpractice for using amalgam and suspended them.

Over the second half of the nineteenth century, the question of amalgam safety was debated fiercely. By the turn of the century, however, with mass production and the significantly lower cost of mercury than gold fillings, mercury amalgams were being placed routinely despite warnings from scientists. Dr. Alfred Stock, a German scientist, published many articles before World War II warning about the dangers of mercury amalgams.[3] Commercial interests clearly had influenced the dental industry to such a degree that dentists chose to ignore the well-documented dangers of mercury. In the 1980s, however, Dr. Hal Huggins ignited the mercury amalgam controversy in the United States once again. Then, in 1989, the EPA declared that mercury amalgams are a hazardous substance under the Superfund Law.[4] As this issue began to receive publicity, it unleashed a furious battle between the American television media and the dental profession. The media accused the dental profession of endangering their patients' health, and the American Dental Association vehemently denied that mercury in amalgams is unsafe. Today, in the midst of this hotly debated issue, the American Dental Association continues to state that the amount of mercury released from mercury amalgam dental fillings does not present a health hazard except in those individuals who are allergic to mercury. The U.S. government has not stepped in to moderate this issue, but governments of many other industrialized nations disagree with the American Dental Association's position. Norway, Sweden, Germany, Denmark, Austria, Finland, and Canada are taking action to protect their citizens. All of these countries have legislated limiting and phasing out the use of dental amalgam restorations.[5]

These silver fillings, as the dental profession called them for decades, are, in fact, a mixture of mercury, silver, copper, tin, zinc, and nickel. Mercury is the major component of new amalgam fillings, at 52 percent. Over time this mercury leaches out of our fillings into our mouths. One study found that the 52 percent mercury content of new amalgams is reduced to 37 percent mercury after five years. On average, one amalgam filling weighs 1 g and contains 0.5 g of mercury. The typical adult carries ten amalgam fillings containing about 5 g of mercury. Half a gram of mercury in a ten-acre lake, under current environmental laws, would warrant an advisory of fish contamination for the entire lake.[6]

Equally worrisome is the fact that mercury in our amalgams gives off methylmercury vapors. Methylmercury is considered to be the most dangerous of all the mercury compounds. Unlike inorganic mercury, methylmercury is a poison that is extremely subtle, difficult to detect, and long-lasting. It is bound by hemoglobin in the red blood cells and passes easily into the central nervous system, where it irreversibly damages the cells of the cerebellum, the cerebral cortex, and the calcarine cortex.[7] The newer the amalgam filling, the more methylmercury vapor is emitted. Researchers have found very high levels of mercury vapor in the mouths of people who chew gum. The chewing action releases vapors from their mercury amalgams. And, since heat also acts on the amalgams, eating hot food and drinking hot liquids also will prompt a rise in the level of mercury vapor in the mouth. This mercury vapor is toxic and can provoke a complex set of symptoms, including neurologic damage.[8]

There is evidence that mercury may play a role in the pathogenesis of brain tumors. Results of many epidemiologic studies indicate that there is a "much higher incidence of brain tumors among urban people in the Western, industrialized world than among more primitive and rural populations."[9] Native American, native Hawaiian, and African rural populations, who tend to have excellent teeth and, therefore, little or no dental treatment with mercury amalgams, have a very low rate of brain tumors.

After I had acquired this general knowledge of problems with mercury amalgams, I decided to look for specific scientific research data to verify the sorts of health problems mercury amalgam could effect. By this time I strongly suspected that my autoimmune illness could be linked to my dental work. I include some of these research findings here to point out the inherent dangers of mercury amalgams for you as a lupus patient. Let's look first at some general psychological problems associated with mercury amalgams.

In one study of the symptoms of forty-seven patients with mercury amalgams compared with those of forty-eight patients without amalgam in their teeth, the people with amalgam were found to experience less happiness and less peace of mind, and had poorer reading ability as well as a higher prevalence of foul breath, tremors, colds and respiratory infections, heart or chest pains, heartburn, menstrual difficulties, sudden anger, depression, irritability, tiring easily, morning fatigue, hay fever, trouble with night vision, and metallic taste in the mouth. The lead researcher in the study states, "Most of these symptoms can be explained by mercury toxicity."[10]

In another study done on twenty-five women with amalgams and twenty-three women without amalgams, researchers found that women with amalgams had statistically significantly more symptoms of fatigue and insomnia as well as more episodes of anger without provocation. They had higher anxiety levels and were less satisfied, less happy, less secure, less steady, and less able to make difficult decisions. The study suggests that amalgam mercury may be a causal factor in depression, excessive anger, and anxiety.[11]

Now let's look at the way mercury affects the immune response, possibly bringing about SLE and other autoimmune diseases. A brief microbiology lesson may help us understand this extremely important material. We have a nonspecific immune response that reacts to inflammation and heals it. We also have a specific or "acquired" immune response that is more complex. The warriors of our defense system are the white blood cells, called *leukocytes* that destroy alien invaders in our system, such as bacteria and viruses. Another group of white blood cells termed *lymphocytes* identify these invaders as different from our own natural cells and body chemicals.

Some lymphocytes, the B cells, produce antibodies in response to a specific antigen (such as bacteria). These antibodies, members of a larger group of blood proteins called immunoglobulins, circulate through the bloodstream and act alone or with natural killer (NK) lymphocytes to neutralize or destroy the antigens. Another type of lymphocyte, the T cell, exists in two different forms. The helper T CD4 cells identify foreign invaders, which can be pathogens or chemicals, distinguish them from our own body tissue, and initiate the immune defense response by activating other lymphocytes, such as B cells and suppressor T CD8 cells. The T CD8 cells, in turn, kill the targeted foreign cells. It is critically important that the helper T CD4 cells maintain their ability to distinguish foreign materials from the body's own tissue and that the suppressor T CD8 cells preserve their capacity to complete the response.

Many of us with lupus understand that our immune responses are confused, attacking our own tissue because it appears to be foreign material. This happens when our T cells are damaged and become unable to identify our body substances as "self." Moreover, a foreign invader, such as a chemical, may attach to our own normal body tissue. For example, mercury can attach to the sulfur atom of a body protein. If this happens, the T CD4 cells no longer can recognize the body's protein as "self," and the T CD8 cells move in to attack and destroy. This catapults us into allergic reactions. If the insult persists over time, we can slide into the abyss of chronic autoimmune disease.[12]

Methylmercury can wreak havoc on the human body. In 1987 Swedish scientists established that mercury vapor from amalgam load leads to mercury accumulation in the tissues of the brain and kidneys.[13] Subsequent research established that mercury affects the hemoglobin level. With more amalgam in our teeth, our blood appears to carry less hemoglobin. At the same time, the leukocytes that we need to fight disease are extremely sensitive to mercury changes in our body; the more mercury is present, the lower the white cell count will be. This has led researchers to suspect that mercury makes us more susceptible to such diseases as cancer and AIDS.[14] Another highly regarded study states that there is evidence that mercury in dental amalgams can lower the T-lymphocyte count, resulting in weakening of the immune system. The conclusion this researcher drew from this unsettling study was that "an abnormal T-lymphocyte percent . . . or a malfunction of T lymphocytes can increase the risk of cancer, infectious diseases, and autoimmune diseases."[15]

In 1970, researchers at the University of Oregon Medical School reported in a landmark study that low doses of inorganic and organic mercury altered lymphocytes in humans who had a demonstrated allergy to mercury.[16] Other researchers found in 1980 that 90 percent of rats exposed to low doses of inorganic mercury had mercury-induced antinuclear antibodies, meaning that the antibodies attacked the nuclei of the rats' cells. The presence of these antinuclear antibodies is one of the primary screening criteria for determining whether a person has lupus. The rats in the study also showed a significant impairment of stimulation of lymphocytes, meaning that they would be less able to respond to an immune challenge.[17]

In 1982, another study found that autoimmune disease caused by mercury could affect the kidneys, spleen, intestine, liver, lung, and heart. All forms of mercury could trigger autoimmune disease, whether it was through inhalation, vapors from amalgam fillings, or intravenous (through the vein), subcutaneous (injected under the skin), or percutaneous (absorbed through the skin) introduction to the human body.[18] More recent research continues to show that amalgam and nickel impair the helper T cell and suppressor T cell. A low T4/T8 ratio can predispose us to autoimmune diseases, such as SLE, hemolytic anemia, multiple sclerosis, severe atopic eczema, inflammatory bowel disease, and kidney disease.[19]

Another study gave strong indications that dental amalgam toxicity may provoke immune system overreactivity. The chemistry of this effect lies in the fact that mercury binds to various organ proteins that the immune system "reads" as foreign substance. That chain reaction elicits an "autoaggressive response," which is the essence of autoimmune disease.[20] More alarming connections between mercury and autoimmune disease come from a controlled study of mice. Some strains of mice with a genetic predisposition to immune imbalance are highly susceptible to mercury-induced autoimmunity. Treatment with mercury chloride induces systemic autoimmune disease in certain mice and rats, which takes the form of production of antinuclear antibodies.[21]

As if this attack on our own immune systems from mercury amalgams weren't enough, an elegantly designed animal study in the late 1980s proved that mercury in the mother's teeth was absorbed by the fetus. Mercury from dental amalgams placed in pregnant ewes appeared in maternal and fetal blood and the fluid of the amnion (the sac containing the embryo) within two days after placement in the mother's teeth. Excretion of some of this mercury also commenced within two days. Although all tissues were affected, the highest concentrations in the fetus appeared in the liver and pituitary gland. The researchers concluded that mercury vapor released from dental amalgam fillings is absorbed readily into the lungs, gastrointestinal tract, and jawbone and progressively accumulates in maternal and fetal tissues with longer durations of exposure. Mercury exposure from this dental material occurs in the newborn baby via the mother's milk. The authors of the study stated that, "our laboratory findings in this investigation are at variance with the anecdotal opinion of the dental profession, which claims that amalgam tooth fillings are safe."[22] This study suggests that those of us born to mothers with mercury amalgams already had mercury in our tissues as fetuses and newborns.

There is more recent evidence that a mother's mercury amalgams affect the fetus. In a European study conducted in 1994, liver and kidney autopsy specimens from 108 children, aged one day to five years, were examined for mercury concentrations in tissue. The research report states that the concentration of mercury in the liver of fetuses was significantly associated with the number of amalgam fillings in the mother. Researchers reporting this finding strongly advocated stopping the use of dental amalgams in women before and during childbearing years.[23] These two research studies led the Swedish government to ban, on February 18, 1994, the placement of mercury amalgams in pregnant women and children under nineteen years of age, because evidence showed these amalgams to be a trigger for autoimmune disorders.[24]

Finally, another alarming Swedish research report on mercury amalgam is important for those of us who spend many hours at our computers. Scientists are aware that some people have a higher rate of mercury absorption from their amalgam fillings than other people, but they've been mystified as to the reasons for this phenomenon.[25] This Swedish study documented that sitting in front of computer screens containing cathode ray tubes sets up a magnetic field that significantly amplifies the release of mercury vapor from the amalgams in the mouth of the computer operator.[26] Since reading that study, I have been shopping for a laptop computer with a liquid crystal display screen, which is far safer than the cathode ray tube of conventional computer monitors. Television screens also contain cathode ray tubes. Since we generally sit farther away from them than we do from computer screens, the magnetic fields produced by TV screens may be less dangerous than those produced by computers.

If we have our amalgams removed, can we get well? There are five disease categories that may be helped by amalgam removal—neurologic, cardiovascular, collagen, immunologic, and allergy. Evidence now exists that sequential removal of dental amalgams can produce remission of many disease symptoms and improve blood chemistry, urinary excretion of mercury, blood pressure, and body temperature. It also can improve results of electrocardiograms, vision and retinal change, and blood circulation to the brain.[27]

Of great relevance for us as lupus patients is the fact that collagen disease may be reversed with removal of amalgam fillings. Dr. Huggins mentions lupus erythematosus and scleroderma as well as arthritis as possibly amenable to dental amalgam removal. One patient came to him with arthritis and a "tentative" diagnosis of SLE. He found negative electrical current on a nickel crown in her mouth. Methylmercury is more apt to appear in the mouth in the presence of a negative current. Two months after her amalgams and crowns were removed, she could use her hands again, stopped stuttering, regained her memory, and lost her paranoia.[28]

In addition to anecdotal accounts, there is scientific evidence that people who are ill may feel better with amalgam removal. One Swedish study indicated that immune parameters improve after amalgam removal. Fifty-three patients with complaints they attributed to their amalgam fillings, and with tests results showing abnormality of their immune systems, were followed for one to three years after the removal of all, some, or none of their amalgam fillings. Within the group of thirty-four individuals who had all their amalgam fillings replaced, there was a statistically significant number who showed decreased antibody counts, which was a positive development. Moreover, a significant improvement in a number of the patients' subjective symptoms occurred in 59 percent of the cases. The researchers concluded, "It thus seems that mercury released from amalgam fillings may initiate or support an ongoing immune disease."[29]

Reading all this material was enough to convince me that I needed to have my amalgams removed. Although I dreaded the procedures involved in extracting twenty-two mercury amalgams, all requiring use of the rubber dam that makes it difficult to breath and swallow, I knew I needed to go through the procedure. Equally worrisome for me was the fact that I had become so chemically sensitive that I feared I might react to the dental anesthetic. Another problem was finding a dentist in our conservative city who believed in the dangers of mercury amalgams. Luck was with me. By networking, I found a young dentist who agreed that the methylmercury from my amalgams could be contributing to my illness. He had received special training in removing mercury amalgams, and he was willing to order a special anesthetic that he thought I could tolerate. This pleasant man also agreed to replace my mercury amalgams with dental materials identified as safe for me using sensitivity tests performed at a laboratory in

Colorado. During the preparatory phase, I learned that amalgams can be replaced with bonded resins—composites made of ground glass powder mixed with a plastic binder. But not everyone can tolerate these materials. People who are extremely chemically sensitive may fare better with gold fillings rather than bonded resins.

At this time I also worked with a hypnotherapist to prepare for enduring the dental procedures. I was so weak and fatigued from my lupus, that I wondered whether I could make it through the dental restorations. To move beyond my dread, with the help of the hypnotherapist, I began to practice mentally leaving the dentist's chair and clinic, going elsewhere with my thoughts when the drilling and probing began to feel intolerable.

At my first appointment, the dentist used a machine called an *amalgameter* to detect negative electrical current on my teeth. Negative current is associated closely with neurologic problems, both muscular (as with multiple sclerosis) and emotional. An amalgameter reading can be used to determine positive and negative charges in the fillings. Then, if the negatively charged fillings are removed first, starting with those generating the highest readings, the patient's chances of health improvements are good. More specifically, if all the fillings are removed first from the quadrant (one-fourth of the mouth) with the highest negative readings, the patient will have an 80 percent chance of getting well. This procedure is extremely important, because people cannot recover if it is not followed.

My dental work began with the dentist first sequentially removing the amalgams in the quadrant with the highest electrical readings. Reclining in the dentist's chair, masked with a rubber dam, and knowing the dentist was using a water spray drill and high-volume vacuum evacuator to protect me from the mercury that was being drilled, I knew that I didn't want to be there. I moved out of my body, using the hypnosis training, and went off to visit the ocean beaches I had loved as a child. One day, during a particularly difficult and lengthy dental drilling procedure, I returned to the high savanna where I had lived in East Africa, spending time with the elephant herds. Other days, when I thought I could not endure another second of drilling, I went off to visit the lovely gardens my husband and I had created.

During one procedure I mentally designed a new herb garden. Another dental appointment found me in the chair constructing the small solar house of my dreams.

Because we had to proceed slowly—often waiting weeks before we removed and replaced another filling so that my weakened body could recover—the amalgam replacements went on for more than a year and a half. By that time we had replaced seventeen fillings, leaving five with low electrical currents. During that time my energy level slowly improved, and my motor control returned so that I did not have to hang on to sofas and walls to walk. My gums also began to heal. One morning shortly after the dentist removed one of my old crowns, I had the sudden urge to urinate. I signaled the dental assistant that I needed to leave the chair and rushed to the restroom. During the next twenty-four hours I urinated more than forty times. About two weeks later, according to my journals, I noticed that I began to perspire when I was trudging uphill on my daily walk. I had not been able to perspire in years. Many of us with lupus have kidney problems. Now I realized that my edema, which had plagued me for more than ten years, was finally correcting and that my kidneys were strengthening. All of these physical improvements were a sign that my body was moving back into balance.

When I asked the dentist which metal had lined the old crown he replaced, he said it was nickel. I recalled the woman with lupus and a nickel crown who improved when the crown was removed, according to Dr. Huggins. I knew I had a nickel allergy; I could not wear costume jewelry or sandals with metal buckles—all of which contain nickel—owing to the burning, oozing skin rash it caused. Could the nickel in that crown have brought about my nickel allergy? And could that nickel in my mouth be contributing to my lupus? I strongly suspected this was the case.

SHOULD YOU CONSIDER HAVING YOUR AMALGAMS REMOVED?

Scientific documentation has established that mercury causes dysfunction of the immune system as well as autoimmune disease itself. I'm sure you will agree that the implications of the scientific studies on mercury amalgam are very serious for those of us with lupus. To help you decide whether you might need to have your dental amalgams removed, think back over your health history, looking for a connection between your health status and placement of dental materials in your mouth. Can you correlate the onset of lupus symptoms with any dental work? If you think you can, having your amalgams removed and your crowns replaced with gold or pure porcelain (no metal liners), would be a positive step, but only if you're strong enough to endure the stress of the dental work.

It is critical that you work with a dentist who has been trained to remove dental amalgams sequentially and have those fillings replaced with materials that blood tests verify your system can tolerate. You'll need to look carefully into the costs and whether your dental insurance will cover the restorative work. Proceed with caution, however, because some dentists who perform these procedures call themselves specialists and charge exorbitant fees. Many other dentists are honest and reasonable in their fees. Look for a dentist who operates a mercury-free practice and understands your need to have your fillings removed and replaced with nonmetallic fillings.

Be aware that in the current climate of hostility, dentists must be careful of what they say to their patients about mercury amalgams. Should your dentist tell you about the dangers of methylmercury, he or she could be disciplined by the American Dental Association.[30] If you are unable to find a dentist in your geographic area who is trained in specific mercury removal and replacement techniques, see the resource section at the back of this book for referrals to dentists in your area who have completed this training. Meanwhile, as you're informing yourself about the dangers of mercury amalgams, how can you take care of yourself? There are two immediate steps you can take. First, refuse to allow any dentist to place more mercury amalgam in your teeth. Second, stop chewing gum, because it has been shown to release mercury vapor from your fillings, which then is absorbed into your body.

There are ways to neutralize in part the effects of mercury toxicity in your body. Clinical evidence suggests that a selenium deficiency enhances the symptoms of mercury poisoning.[31] Therefore, selenium can have a neutralizing effect on mercury toxicity. Selenium binds with mercury and will start to effect a redistribution of mercury in your tissue. Take a 50-mg tablet of selenium three times a day with each meal. Start the selenium slowly if you are chemically sensitive, so that you can avoid an adverse reaction.

Another important mineral is magnesium. It is essential for the functioning of several hundred enzymes in the body. The presence of mercury depresses metabolic functions of magnesium, and, for this reason, it is critically important to take this supplement if you have amalgams in your mouth.[32] Take one 100-mg tablet at bedtime.[33]

It is advisable to start taking the amino acid glutathione, 50 mg three times a day on an empty stomach, which will provide some protection against mercury damage. Zinc can help the body detoxify the effects of mercury. Take 15 to 30 mg once a day. Finally, you should take one 50-mg tablet of vitamin B_1 (thiamine) with each meal (for a total of 150 mg per day) and 15 to 25 mg of B complex each day.[34] It is important to take large doses of B_1 because it can strengthen the immune system. Taken in conjuction with smaller doses of B complex, it can also protect the nervous system.

You may start to feel better in three to five days, or it may take sixty to ninety days. You may not feel any better at all. Following this regimen, I felt somewhat better and was encouraged to think seriously about amalgam removal. I continued to follow this plan for the duration of the restorative procedures, to help my body detoxify from any mercury burdens caused by the removal process.

You also can make dietary changes to lower mercury levels in your system. Consider eating less fish or no fish, since it is the largest dietary source of mercury. Stop eating shellfish, because they are scavengers and may contain high levels of heavy metals. Increase your fiber intake by eating more vegetables. Drink six to eight glasses of water a day, which will help rid your body of toxins. Take psyllium husk in water, which will bind with heavy metals in your body and remove them. Eat unsweetened yogurt with live cultures, kefir, or acidophilus supplements, which will assist in maintaining your intestinal flora.

There is another way to eliminate the heavy metal toxicity that may result from mercury amalgam removals. You can use chelation therapy before or after each dental appointment, to remove the mercury that is released in the amalgam removal process. The chelating agent EDTA (synthesized amino acid disodium) binds with mercury and then is excreted in the urine and feces.[35] Chelation therapy must be done under the supervision of a licensed medical doctor. Physicians who are aware of the adverse role of heavy metals in the human body generally belong to the American College of Advancement in Medicine. Some of them acknowledge the mercury amalgam problem. Be sure to verify that the physician you use is board certified in chelation therapy. You also can use oral chelating agents, which only recently have come on the market. Talk with your alternative health care provider about trying this oral chelation method as a less invasive and less expensive method for removing mercury from your system.

At the end of seventeen amalgam removals and one crown replacement, I stopped the dental work to take a much needed rest. The work had been expensive, but our dental plan had paid half the cost. I have subsequently had the rest of my amalgam fillings removed and am pleased to report that I am now free of mercury in my mouth. My energy level continued to improve as my kidney and bladder functions strengthened. I could think more clearly again, and my burning eyes and dry throat disappeared. Finally, my feeling of "burning up inside," which I had experienced for more than ten years, began to resolve.

This most arduous journey of my twelve-year search for wellness had succeeded. After identifying and freeing my body from the most toxic non-radioactive compound on earth, I felt confident that I was finally recovering my health at the deepest level. Exhausted from the stress of this last safari through hostile terrain, I released my faithful camels to the desert. Then, hoisting my dusty packs and tattered journals, I hiked home to rest before I continued my journey.

10

Traditional Chinese Medicine

In transposing Chinese ideas into our own idiom, our challenge has been to bridge gaps—between mind and body, theory and practice, therapy and self-care, practitioner and patient, ancient and modern, convention and invention, East and West. Through cultural blending, we are transmuting wisdom from early China into what has relevance for us today.

Harriet Beinfield, L.Ac., and Efrem Korngold, L.Ac., O.M.D.

During my years of living with lupus, many of my symptoms have been minimized or relieved with various alternative therapies. But dizziness, fatigue, mild depression, and sporadic anxiety continued to plague me. As I searched for an approach that could calm me and improve my mood and energy level, an acquaintance mentioned a woman in California whose lupus had been successfully treated by TCM. Knowing nothing about acupuncture and Chinese herbs at that time, I quickly located books and articles on the subject. The TCM texts revealed a fascinating medical discipline with a written system of acupuncture more than two thousand years old. The practice of acupuncture and use of Chinese herbs is even more ancient—going back at least five thousand years.

My own experience with Oriental medicine has convinced me that this system has great potential for healing SLE. You're probably wondering, as I did, about the healing concepts upon which TCM is based. More specifically, it is important to understand how acupuncture and Chinese herbs work. What are those needles doing? Do they hurt? Will the treatment help me feel any better? Is the procedure safe? Can acupuncture truly treat my lupus? Are traditional Chinese herbal formulas safe? Where can I buy them? These and many more questions arise when we enter a treatment program that is so radically different from conventional Western medicine.

Acupuncture and herbal medicine form a refined system of medical theory and practice. The underlying goal is to create total well-being in the patient. From the TCM viewpoint, acupuncture fine-tunes the interactions of subtle energies in our body. By increasing the chi, acupuncture assists us in self-healing. Chi is defined variously as *energy, vitality, life force,* and *breath.* Strong chi creates lively, energetic people. In contrast, lack of sufficient chi weakens a person. When we are ill, our chi is depleted, bringing on fatigue and depression. Moreover, if our chi is disturbed, we may become irritable and overreactive to situations.

Classical Chinese acupuncture embraces the concept that a subtle system moves chi through the body in a network of channels or meridians. When these channels become blocked, an imbalance occurs, which can be corrected by stimulating points along the meridian. The acupuncturist is trained to take a complex reading of many pulses to check the flow of chi. These pulses have such names as *floating pulse, sinking pulse, thin pulse,* and *empty pulse.* Pulse readings help the acupuncturist determine at which meridian points on the body to place needles to restore the balance of chi, thereby improving both our physical and mental health.[1]

To help us better understand this medical system, the Chinese use the metaphor of the body as a musical instrument constantly resonating with the flow of chi through the meridians as a flute vibrates from a breath of air.

Complete health, from the ancient Chinese perspective, is like a pure, clear note from the flute. Illness, on the other hand, is discord. It can be corrected by stimulating different points on the body, which changes the quality of the chi just as fingering different holes on the flute changes the quality of the musical note.[2]

An interesting ancient concept of TCM states that acupuncture deals with two different environments: the internal and the external. One surrounds us, and the other is contained inside us. Both of these environments have an impact on us. The atmospheric environment consists of the seasonal changes of our weather, in the form of wind, rain, heat, cold, dryness, and dampness. Our internal environment comprises our organs, body fluids, and reproductive functions as well as our thoughts and emotions. Adverse effects from one or both of these environments can provoke illness. On the other hand, if our bodies can manage these negative effects efficiently, we are able to stay well. Acupuncture helps balance the climate of our personal environment with our reactions to the outside environment, which in turn helps us stay healthy.[3]

TCM also uses the concepts of yin and yang, which must be in balance for us to stay well. Yin could be said to refer to the tissue of our organs and yang to the energy in the organs. A yin deficiency would mean that we don't have enough materials to build a strong organ. A yang deficiency, on the other hand, would imply that the organ does not have the energy to perform adequately. The yin and yang systems are interdependent and mirror each other.[4] In general, if one system is disrupted, the other will be out of balance as well.

Once I understood some of the holistic medical theories upon which TCM is based, I called the woman in California whose lupus had responded to TCM treatment. During phone conversations over the next few weeks, Joan told me her story. In the 1960s, when her illness was diagnosed, people with severe lupus were told that there was little help conventional medicine could offer other than glucocorticoids to reduce the inflammation triggered by the autoimmune reaction. Joan also was told that she probably never would recover from lupus. Concerned about the adverse effects of the drugs then being used to treat SLE, she decided to forgo steroids and instead set out looking for another approach.

So ill she could barely walk, Joan somehow managed to drive herself to San Francisco's Asian district to meet a TCM doctor who had recently emigrate from Taiwan. Standing in his tiny store lined with jars of dried apothecary ingredients, she watched the doctor measuring herbs and writing directions for patients in Chinese. He spoke very little English, and she spoke no Cantonese or Mandarin. "Well," Joan thought, "this isn't going to be easy, but I want to try it." Using his wife as an interpreter, the doctor told her that Chinese medical personnel knew about lupus. He said that he had specific herbs and knew the right acupuncture points to try to treat her lupus symptoms.

And so Joan embarked on a journey into TCM. On some days, after acupuncture treatment, she felt much better. On other days she felt significantly worse. Some of the Chinese herbal formulas the doctor created for her relieved her symptoms, and some made her sicker. But she persisted with the treatments, journeying through what was sometimes rough territory, hoping for alleviation of her symptoms.

Finally, after many months of treatment, Joan began to feel increasingly better. The improvements in her health were subtle but concrete. First she could walk a little. Then she could cook a meal occasionally. Later she was able to return to the portrait painting at which she is so skilled. Although her five children grew up during her years of illness, once her health improved, Joan was able to be an active family member again. Entering graduate school after the age of sixty, today she works as a psychologist specializing in geriatric care. Joan's remarkable determination to explore TCM when she was so ill, and when few Americans knew anything about it, has brought her many rewards.

Inspired by Joan's story, I wondered whether TCM might help me regain complete health. Would these ancient teachings have anything to offer in treating my lupus? The answer came in the form of recurring dreams in which my camel caravan undulated over mountain and plateau, slowly transporting Chinese herbal medicines and bundles of tiny needles wrapped in papyrus along the ancient silk road running from China to the Near East. In smoky, parched villages along that ancient caravan route I saw people healing from the medicines and acupuncture. With those images in my mind, I decided to find a TCM practitioner and proceed with treatment. Although there were no TCM practitioners in our small city, after much networking, we found a TCM doctor from China who was teaching and studying at Bastyr University in Seattle. He was hoping to learn how to integrate alternative Western medicine with TCM.

Dr. Cao knew about lupus. During his initial examination, I was surprised to find that he drew no blood and ordered no laboratory tests or radiographs. Instead, he carefully looked at my complexion and my tongue, listened to my voice, smelled my body for odor, and took many pulses at my wrists and ankles. He told me that the TCM diagnosis for my condition was kidney yin deficiency, spleen chi deficiency, and liver chi stagnation. He said that TCM is an excellent system for treating long-term, chronic illness and that he was willing to try to alleviate my symptoms. He also said that, in his opinion, many of the traditional treatments for lupus would be too strong for me because I was so ill and that he would be as gentle with the treatments as possible.

When I asked him how TCM would differ from Western medicine in its treatment of my lupus, Dr. Cao explained that whereas Western medicine generally addresses a specific illness, TCM addresses symptoms in a particular patient and treats the way the patient is responding to the disease, not just the disease itself. I later learned that many TCM doctors speak in metaphors about the body's flows of energy and fluids, as though they are rivers or lakes. TCM practitioners also talk about the elements of wind, heat, cold, dryness, and dampness that the patient might be manifesting in the form of symptoms.

Before I decided to proceed with Dr. Cao's treatment, I arranged a discussion with Anne Christiansen, a licensed acupuncturist and adjunct professor at the Department of Oriental Medicine, Bastyr University, in Seattle. She also has a private acupuncture practice in the Seattle area. I asked her what my diagnoses of kidney yin deficiency, spleen chi deficiency, and liver chi stagnation meant in Western terms. Here is how she explained these to me:

> When a lupus patient goes for TCM, the practitioner first acknowledges the diagnosis and finds out about the Western medications, if any, the lupus patient is taking. Then we begin looking for *patterns*, a key concept in TCM, which is defined by the patient's physical appearance, appearance of the tongue, and the pulse—all of which can be affected by the internal conditions and medications. We aren't looking for illness as much as for disharmony and using specific approaches to recreate harmony.
>
> The important concept here is that we are trained to view each patient as unique, so ten patients with a Western diagnosis of lupus may show ten slightly to significantly different patterns of imbalance and disharmony. We TCM doctors ask, probe, try to find the patterns. Is there too much yin? Is there too much yang? Is the patient drying up? Patients with lupus may show kidney yin deficiency or spleen chi deficiency, but these are very general patterns. The TCM practitioner must step outside those patterns and look at the particulars of that diagnosis, so that he or she can look for the patterns within patterns. With lupus there are patterns specific to the kidney, which may have to do with genetics, with the family history. These are points on the kidney meridian, which is a whole energy field in itself.
>
> In Western medicine we are firmly fixed in cause and effect, but in TCM, practitioners don't wait to see the illness itself develop. We are trained to say, "Let's not wait." This is Taoist-based medicine. We believe that our bodies are the microcosms in the macrocosm. Everything is part of the whole, embracing the patterns of the whole. In TCM we don't treat symptoms so much as we look for the root cause of the imbalance or disharmony.[5]

From my research I learned more about how TCM views and treats lupus. Given the likelihood that we were born with a genetic propensity for the disease, many of us wonder what factors brought on our lupus. Conventional Western medicine says that it doesn't know what causes lupus, but at least one creative TCM clinician, M. M. Van Benschoten, believes that low-grade infection is the culprit. "The failure of both Western and Chinese medicine to adequately address the issue of subclinical infection as the root cause of auto-immune disease [should be corrected]."[6] He states that subclinical infection can be found by applying the "yin–yang vector test of acupoints." This test measures certain spectra of light emissions from acupuncture points to detect the presence of pathogens, quantify their intensity, and test for appropriate medications. Van Benschoten says that, based on the acupoint test, accurately prescribed Chinese herbal formulas can remove the infection, bringing long periods of complete remission of autoimmune symptoms.[7] Some of us also know that the way we live and eat can amplify or minimize our lupus symptoms. TCM identifies the factors that deplete kidney yin—a condition of autoimmune disease—as stress, sex, emotional upset, menstruation, chocolate, sweets, alcohol, coffee, and drugs.[8]

SLE is an extremely complex illness. Interestingly, the Chinese system of diagnosis reflects this complexity. TCM states that autoimmune illness results from a harmful climate inside the body accompanying stagnation of blood and chi. Our fatigue, lethargy, and anemia result from initial heat in the lungs, leading to deficiencies of the kidney and liver.[9] Our hot, inflamed joints, butterfly rashes, mucosal ulcers, and kidney and bladder infections, on the other hand, are signs of excess or disturbed chi and blood.[10] This seeming contradiction between "deficient " and "excess" is what I believe renders Western conventional medicine unable to treat SLE successfully without using powerful, potentially debilitating pharmaceuticals. Because the Western medical view is essentially linear and one dimensional, it seems unable to conceive of illness as circular and multileveled. Since ancient times, TCM has been comfortable with this multidimensional image of illness, which renders it able to treat the complexities of chronic illness from many perspectives.

Any disorder of the immune system, according to TCM, affects the kidneys, which supply the lungs with the vigor needed to create immune energy and distribute it through the blood vessels and meridians to our cells. TCM also maintains that lupus involves deficient lung energies. Treatment focuses on strengthening kidney and lung chi, supporting kidney and lung yin, and dispersing the "raging fires" in the blood, which may cause those of us with lupus to exhibit severe central nervous system symptoms, such as seizures or psychotic episodes.[11] All of this is done using specific acupuncture points and TCM herbal remedies.

During my weekly appointments with Dr. Cao, the tiny needles inserted just under my skin on certain meridian points at first increased my anxiety, but soon I began to feel less frightened of them. Assuring me that the needles are sterilized and disposable, he said there is no danger of contamination. Dr. Cao sometimes teased me, saying, " Today, sixteen needles. When you get to twenty-four needles, then you'll be really important." And we would both laugh. Often I felt much better for a few days after the treatment. Sometimes I felt even more tired and nervous. The doctor also prescribed herbal remedies in conjunction with the acupuncture treatments. At times I felt better taking the herbs; at other times I felt dizzier and more fatigued. After about three months of treatment, my dizziness and fatigue finally began to diminish. I was able to ride in a car more easily, and I could walk half a mile without being exhausted. Slowly, my mild depression lifted, and I became calmer. Deeply grateful for my improving health, Steve and I began to hope that I might someday recover enough to have a stimulating, active life again. Then Dr. Cao moved his practice two hours away, and I was unable to manage the four-hour round trip to visit him.

TCM and the Specific Treatment of Lupus

While I waited for another TCM practitioner to come into my life, I began to examine clinical studies on the efficacy of TCM for treating lupus. During this search I found some heartening information. Ted Kaptchuk, Doctor of Oriental Medicine, describes studies documenting the success of Chinese medicine in treating SLE. Two studies, the first dealing with 120 cases of lupus and the second with twenty-two cases, both concluded that traditional herbal treatments lowered the mortality rates from lupus more effectively than Western therapy and that in a high proportion of cases, Chinese medicine is very helpful in treating the disorder.[12]

Another study, this one conducted by clinicians in 1985 at Shanghai First Medical College on patients with lupus, showed that acupuncture may help people with lupus. I describe this study in some detail to illustrate the dramatic results of acupuncture. Group I, made up of ten patients, manifested skin lesions, joint pain, and mild kidney symptoms. The average age of the all-female group was 29.1 years. The average disease duration was 3.2 years. None of the patients had received glucocorticoids or immunosuppressive drugs. Acupuncture alone was used. Group II, made up of fifteen patients, had nephrotic syndrome (blood chemistry imbalance marked by edema) and had been treated with 50 mg of prednisone daily for five months without improvement. The average age of this group was 23.5 years, and the average disease duration was 3.35 years. Acupuncture was generally used. Group III, comprising twelve patients, had an average age of 29.2 years. They all had lupus nephrotic syndrome for an average disease duration of 4.3 years. This group was treated with glucocorticoids alone.

Patients in groups I and II received acupuncture three times weekly. Two groups of acupuncture points were used interchangeably. For the most part, two courses of ten treatments each were given, for a total of twenty treatments. The doctors carried out follow-up examinations of each group every two weeks for more than six months. Improvement was significant in groups I and II after treatment. Fatigue, low-grade fever, skin lesions, joint pain, and amenorrhea (absence of menstrual flow) were markedly alleviated. In two patients, Raynaud's syndrome (abnormal constriction of the arteries of the extremities) stopped after twenty treatments with acupuncture alone. Diuresis (increased excretion of urine) developed, and edema (fluid retention) began to subside ten days after treatment in 75 percent of the patients. Overall improvement was greater in group I than in group II. After acupuncture treatment, immune function improvement in group I was also much better than in group II.

In group II the glucocorticoid dose was lowered gradually at the same time that acupuncture was given. This study indicates that acupuncture can promote T-cell function, resulting in the reduction of both the hyperfunction of B cells and the production of autoantibodies.[13] This study provides stunning evidence that TCM may help many of us with varying degrees of lupus. Other case studies I have read also suggest that TCM can treat SLE effectively.

One more case study, this one from veterinary medicine, is important to note. A 1990 report in the *American Journal of Acupuncture* showed the potential for using a combination of acupuncture and herbs to treat a dog with severe systemic lupus. In this case, Cheryl Schwartz, D.V.M., used herbal combinations of *Panax* ginseng and acupuncture to tonify the dog's chi. Among other capabilities, ginseng can help stimulate appetite and weight gain. Dr. Schwartz also used the plant *Rehmannia* to clean the animal's liver and nourish its blood. *Citrus reticulata* helped regulate the chi, and *Pinellia* assisted in harmonizing the dog's stomach and spleen. Dr. Schwartz asked the dog's owner to massage three acupuncture points at home, and she used needling of acupuncture points on the dog at two-week intervals. She also restricted the dog's diet.

As the treatment continued for four and a half months, the dog steadily improved. Then the dog had a lupus flare-up. Treatment was adjusted, and after one month the dog recovered again. Dr. Schwartz reported that this protocol was effective in treating and controlling a chronic and acute form of SLE in the dog.[14] The procedures and results of this animal case study are important in terms of their possible application to human SLE treatment.

A few months after Dr. Cao moved his clinic, a TCM doctor started a practice in our city. Like Dr. Cao, Dr. Bing Zhou was also from China and also had been trained in both TCM and conventional Western medicine. This background gave her the ability to synthesize Western medical diagnoses with TCM patterns to create her treatment plans. During our first appointments, Dr. Bing explained to me that she was giving me gentle acupuncture treatments because I was so sensitive. As the weekly treatments progressed, I knew that I was feeling calmer and more rested. But when I returned home from an acupuncture treatment one afternoon and vacuumed three rooms of my house I realized that I was dramatically better! I could not recall when I had last been able to vacuum. When I reported this to Dr. Bing, she joked that she did not want to make me so well that I would clean my whole house. As we giggled, I realized that it was the first time I had been able to laugh about my illness in nearly ten years.

Other improvements followed. My eyes and mouth no longer felt as dry, my internal shakiness and feeling of burning up inside slowly subsided, and my general sadness began to disappear. I looked forward to the treatments each week, knowing that I would feel better after the half hour resting in a darkened room with tiny needles inserted in my body. During my treatments, Dr. Bing and I chatted about TCM, and I learned much about this fascinating approach to healing. When Dr. Bing's staff assistant took maternity leave, I accepted the doctor's invitation to assist her in the clinic two hours a day. Unemployed for more than ten years as the result of my illness, I happily became a volunteer, helping introduce patients to the concepts of TCM. Over the weeks that I assisted Dr. Bing, I observed many patients' symptoms improving and became convinced that this ancient system has great efficacy in treating many chronic health problems.

SAFETY OF CHINESE HERBS

In TCM, acupuncture and herbs are known to work synergistically, and, for this reason, it is important for us to understand the use of Chinese herbs. TCM dispenses herbs in two forms—manufactured Chinese patent medicines, and single herbs in combinations that Chinese doctors or pharmacists prescribe. Traditionally, in the Chinese herbal pharmacy, the pharmacist answers questions from the patients and may offer suggestions on which kind of patent medicines to use. Usually the patient pays only for the herbal medicines—not for the consultations. Traditionally the Chinese herbal pharmacy provides services twenty-four hours a day.

Chinese patent medicines are made according to standard herbal formulas in a strictly monitored standard method of production. With a history spanning more than two thousand years, the formulas for some patent medicines used today date from A.D. 200. Are Chinese patent medicines safe for us to use? In fact, there is some controversy about the safety of these products. Daniel J. Wallace, M.D., states in *The Lupus Book* that "some Chinese herbal remedies contain sulfa derivatives and other substances that can trigger allergic reactions in . . . lupus patients."[15]

When I asked Anne Christiansen, licensed acupuncturist and TCM instructor, about the purity and cleanliness of Chinese patent medicines, she had this to say:

> A group of [trained TCM practitioners] is attempting to check the quality and safety of the Chinese formulas. Spot-checks have revealed that there are sometimes Western drugs, such as aspirin or sulfa, in the Chinese preparations. Products from the best Chinese herbal factories are safe, but these production facilities do not seem to be regulated as tightly as are American factories. Some small operations in China produce counterfeit products. The labeling on these products is so good that it's impossible for us to tell them apart.
>
> Many people practicing TCM in this country also are concerned about using preparations that contain parts of animals and plants that are endangered. To address the problems of quality and proper ethics at the source, many TCM practitioners now are using herbal preparations made from herbs that are grown only in this country under strict organic guidelines that contain no animal parts whatsoever.[16]

While we need to acknowledge these potential problems, I believe that it is also important for us to explore Chinese patent medicines, because they have strong potential for helping us recover from lupus. There are other TCM practitioners who think that the major manufacturers of these products in China maintain extremely high standards. The Beijing Tung Jen Tang Pharmacy, for example, is one of the largest in China. Established in 1669, members of the same family have managed the company for more than three hundred years. The manager of Tung Jen Tang says that his companies' patent medicines are superior for three reasons. First, most of their formulas originated from the Imperial Palace and have been observed to be effective over many decades. Second, the herbs used in these formulas are of very high quality and are grown in special geographic areas. Finally, the production process at Tung Jen Tang is monitored strictly for quality control of patent medicines.[17]

Beginning in the 1950s the government of China encouraged increased production of patent medicines as the population rapidly expanded. By the 1970s, production had grown so much that confusion developed over the 6,499 different patent medicines. People were unsure whether all the medicines were being produced according to the ancient formulas in clean, controlled manufacturing environments. To clear up the confusion, the Chinese government decided to regulate the industry in 1985 by issuing the Drug Control Regulations Act. This law is meant to guarantee the quality of drugs manufactured in China and is particularly important for overseas consumers of Chinese patent medicines.

Margaret Naeser, an American Ph.D. and licensed TCM practitioner who spends time in China researching TCM approaches to treating stroke victims, states that this drug control law is being enforced strictly. In the first year after it became effective, the Chinese government destroyed poor-quality or expired medicines and required uncertified patent medicine producers to comply with established standards. In 1986, as a result of this law, several people who were involved in the production and sale of fake medicines were sent to prison. The Chinese government continues to regulate carefully the manufacture of patent medicines.[18] Even with this regulation, however, it's important to work with licensed TCM practitioners in this country who are able to prescribe Chinese patent medicines produced by companies that follow the strictest standards.

CHINESE HERBS FOR TREATING LUPUS

In my research I found two translated clinical studies documenting the efficacy of using specific herbs for treating lupus. One study concluded that six Chinese herbs may improve defective in vitro (outside the living organism) interleukin-2 production in patients with SLE. Interleukin-2 helps increase T-cell counts and enhances natural killer cell functions. This study looked at the in vitro effects of these herbs on mice with genetically inherited lupus. The researchers found that *Codonopsis pilosula* could prolong the life span of female mice with lupus and inhibit antibody production against DNA. *Angelica sinensis* prolonged life spans but did not inhibit the production of DNA antibodies. The researchers stated that these herbs could have great potential for the treatment of human SLE in the future.[19]

Another study also suggested that specific herbs used in TCM can aid in the treatment of lupus. In a research paper published in the *Shanghai Journal of Traditional Chinese Medicine,* clinicians reported that a thirty-two-year-old patient manifesting many lupus symptoms was given a traditional Chinese formula that included *Rehmannia glutinosa, Polygonus multiflorum,* and *Paeonia lactiflora.* This treatment successfully increased the patient's yin energy in the heart, liver, and kidneys, thereby reducing the patient's symptoms.[20]

Chinese patent medicines also have the potential for helping those of us with lupus. Xiao Yo Wan, for example, is a treatment for the liver symptoms many lupus patients exhibit. This formula contains *Radix bupleuri, Radix angelicae sinensis, Radix paeoniae lactiflorae, and Radix glycyrrhizae ivalensis,* among other ingredients. With its capacity to treat liver chi stagnation, this formula is well known historically for diminishing or eliminating symptoms of hypochondria, headache, vertigo, dry mouth and throat, fatigue, poor appetite, moodiness, feeling alternately hot and cold, and menstrual irregularities.[21] I have been helped by this patent medicine and continue to take it because I become slightly dizzy, more fatigued, more nervous, and have more digestive problems when I stop using it.

Yin Qiao Jie Du Pian is another Chinese patent medicine that has helped me and which I believe can help many lupus patients. If used early enough, this medicine can ward off flu, colds, acute bronchitis, and pneumonia. The minute you feel a cold or chills coming on, take three to five coated tablets two to three times a day with warm water. It is important to know that tablet content in these medicines is consistent and standard. The manufacturers of each of these medicines blend from one standard recipe and are not allowed to deviate from it. Continue to take the tablets if you begin to feel better, until the symptoms disappear. If this remedy does not help in three to four days, stop taking it. The active ingredients in this patent medicine include japonica and forsythia, both of which grow in many of our gardens in the Pacific Northwest.

He Che Da Zao Wan, also called *Restorative Pills,* have been recommended to me by a licensed acupuncturist for treating lupus. This formula can address the underlying kidney and lung deficiencies of SLE. In addition to many plants, this medicine contains tortoiseshell and human placenta. Specifically prepared to support kidney, liver, and heart yin functions, this famous remedy also nourishes the blood and treats the "rising fire" inflammation that is so common in lupus. Take eight pills three times daily or twelve pills twice daily until you feel better.[22] Then try stopping the medicine—if your symptoms return, resume taking the pills.

If you do not want to take medicines containing endangered animal parts or human placenta, there is another possibility—Liu Wei Di Huang Wan, or Six Flavor Rehmannia Pills. A classic formula for supporting the yin, particularly kidney yin, it contains six herbs: rehmannia root, cornus fruit, dioscorea root, moutan bark, poria fungus, and alisma root. The TCM prescription is to take eight pills three times a day or twelve pills twice a day. Although this formula helps me feel better in many ways, it also makes me somewhat dizzy, so I take it only occasionally. But I would encourage you to try it for relief of some of your lupus symptoms. Start with half the dose and work up gradually. Stay on this medicine one to two months to give it a chance to work.

In addition to the Chinese patent medicines, you can try taking individual herbs, bearing in mind that the Chinese believe that combinations of herbs are more effective. Rehmannia root, (botanical name, *Rehmannia glutinosa Libosch*) is well known for treating lupus symptoms. The efficacy of this herb lies in its ability to assist at the kidney and liver meridians by toning the blood, minimizing night sweats, protecting the liver, and treating kidney yin deficiency, which includes dizziness and vertigo.[23] I have found rehmannia to be helpful in treating my severe dizziness and vertigo, which kept me from riding in cars or airplanes for more than ten years.

Another helpful single herb is waxtree *(Ligustrum lucidum Ait)*. This plant successfully addresses liver and kidney deficiency by tonifying the kidneys, thus sharpening the vision and alleviating dizziness, ringing in the ears, and heart palpitations. Although I have not used this herb myself, your TCM practitioner may suggest that it is appropriate for treating your symptoms.[24]

One more herb deserves mention here, because it was introduced at the 1992 International Lupus Conference in London as a possible treatment for lupus. It is the Asian shrub *Tripterygium wilfordii*. This traditional Chinese remedy is being used in China today to treat lupus, rheumatoid arthritis, and other autoimmune disorders. It appears to have an anti-inflammatory effect similar to that of glucocorticoids.[25] Western conventional medicine takes the position that this herb needs more research before it is prescribed for the treatment of lupus. TCM, on the other hand, observes that the herb can successfully eliminate or minimize autoimmune symptoms and proceeds with its clinical use. These and hundreds more Chinese patent medicines and herbs are available over the counter at Asian pharmacies. Be sure to consult a licensed TCM practitioner or herbalist before taking any of them for your lupus symptoms.

TCM HOME CARE FOR LUPUS

A small home acupuncture machine I ordered from Australia called the Acuhealth has been of great help to me in minimizing my joint and muscle pain. It uses a blunt needle to allow electrical stimulation of specific acupuncture points. This battery-powered machine comes with an instruction manual keyed to symptoms, with illustrations and written directions. I used it regularly for two years and now use it only occasionally when my pain level rises. Although there are no meridian points listed for lupus, there are points for nervousness, anxiety, depression, dizziness, joint and muscle pain, and fatigue, all of which are symptoms of lupus. The electro-stimulation this machine emits, when applied to appropriate meridian points, has helped with whiplash and shoulder, neck, and joint pain resulting from an auto accident. See the resource section at the end of this book for information on how to order the Acuhealth home acupuncture machine.

Another excellent TCM home care approach is to massage acupressure points that will balance and support chi. For each of these points, use moderate pressure of your thumbs or forefingers, massaging gently in a tiny circle. Try one minute of acupressure on each point twice a day. One good point for lupus is the Conception Vessel 3. At this point, the three yin meridians of the liver, spleen, and kidney intersect the central yin meridian. By working this point, you will increase your healing yin energy and distribute that energy to every organ in your body. This point is located in the center of the lower abdomen about three inches above the pubic bone.

Another helpful meridian point for lupus is Lung 9. This point helps the lung circulate blood and balance the chi. By moving the blood, this point helps the body eliminate excess heat, the cause of such lupus symptoms as rashes and inflamed organs and joints. This point is located on the inside wrist crease below the thumb. Use acupressure on both wrist creases.

An important acupressure point for the kidneys is Kidney 3, which nourishes every kidney point, including the yin, yang, and chi. Because lupus stresses the kidneys, massaging this point can help revive kidney energy. You will find the Kidney 3 point in the depression between your inside ankle bone and your Achilles tendon. Massage this tender spot in a clockwise rotation.[26] Although working these acupressure points will not bring you immediate relief, if you use this self-care approach at least once daily, it will help you over time. For helpful books on acupressure see Suggested Reading at the end of this book.

TRADITIONAL CHINESE FOOD FOR TREATING LUPUS

Another way to help ourselves recover from lupus is to eat foods that can heal us. To the Chinese, food is medicine; there is no separation between the two. Here is a delicious recipe for sautéed chicken and walnuts, used to treat kidney yin deficiency and for warming the lungs.

10 walnuts, halved or quartered
$^1/_2$ to $^3/_4$ cup chopped chicken meat, precooked
5 small pieces black fungus (Chinese dried), soaked and slivered

1 small green chili pepper, minced (optional, depending on your
   digestion)

1 egg white

4 Chinese dried mushrooms, soaked, stemmed, and slivered

1 teaspoon minced scallion

1 clove crushed garlic

1 tablespoon cooking sherry

1 teaspoon soy sauce

$1/_2$ teaspoon salt

$1/_2$ teaspoon honey or sugar

$1/_2$ cup toasted sesame seeds

1 to 2 tablespoons canola oil

Soak the walnuts in hot water until the skins loosen. Peel them and sauté
in oil with the chicken, one scrambled egg white, and the other ingredients.
Sauté for five to seven minutes and serve hot with rice. This takes thirty to
forty minutes to prepare and serves two.[27]

Using these TCM protocols at home can be a great benefit to us. If you
decide to undergo treatment by a TCM practitioner, he or she can give you
many more ideas for acupressure points, gentle exercise, and food combinations that will help you.

THE PRACTICE OF TCM IN THE UNITED STATES

With TCM becoming more available in the United States, we, as health
consumers, need information on how to use this system to help us regain
our health. Here are additional excerpts from my interview with Anne
Christiansen, which address a number of questions many of us who are not
familiar with TCM may have.

Author: Are Americans trained in TCM as good as their Chinese coun-
terparts? What credentials do Americans need? Are people trained in
Taiwan getting a more truly traditional training than people trained in
Mainland China?

Christiansen: Yes, I believe Americans trained in the rigors of TCM can function as effectively as Chinese TCM practitioners. The full TCM program in China takes five years. It is an integration of Western medicine and Oriental medicine, and the graduates are then called *doctors of Oriental medicine*. In Taiwan, students are more classically trained in the real Taoist tradition. In Japan, and even in France, the classic form of TCM has flourished more than it has in modern China with its communist regime, which has not been as sensitive to traditional therapies.

Author: Is acupuncture really effective if done only once a week? In China, I understand they treat every day for two weeks to one month.

Christiansen: Yes, it can be very effective even if it's only once a week. The treatment will be prolonged, and it will take longer to see results, which is actually an acceptable way to treat chronic illness. It would be good to have acupuncture every day for acute conditions.

Author: How can people find licensed TCM practitioners who are trained in all the pulse work and dietary protocols as well as acupuncture and herbs?

Christiansen: The National Certification Commission licenses us when we pass all the required tests. Our training is lengthy and difficult, and we are fully prepared to practice TCM when we acquire our license. Patients need to look for the license in an acupuncture clinic, which should be hanging near the front door.

Author: I believe that TCM could improve our health care system if it were allowed to influence conventional American medicine. Is an integration of Western medicine and TCM occurring anywhere?

Christiansen: Yes! There is an integration of Western medicine and TCM going on in academic settings, especially in clinics, where students are learning TCM and then bringing their own ways of thinking to the techniques. TCM allows this integration, because it is not a rigid system.

Author: Is there any danger for lupus patients being treated with TCM?

Christiansen: The only danger would be malpractice. Patients must check out the licensing of their practitioners. Otherwise, TCM is very safe.

Author: I have found TCM to be very helpful for me. Have you observed lupus patients responding to treatment with TCM?

Christiansen: Yes. This is profound medicine. This is powerful medicine. It can treat deep, difficult illnesses. At Bastyr University clinic, I have seen lupus patients improve. We have even treated HIV-positive patients with TCM and helped them feel better. TCM also can be used with other medical approaches safely and effectively.[28]

FINDING A QUALIFIED ACUPUNCTURIST

TCM has come a long way in this country since the early 1970s when Miriam Lee, an Oriental medical doctor, was arrested in California for performing acupuncture. At her trial hundreds of her patients testified to the help she had given them, protesting that they were being denied their right to choose to be treated with acupuncture. Responding to this public outcry, the California legislature legalized acupuncture as an "experimental procedure" within days of the trial. In 1976 Governor Jerry Brown signed the bill legalizing acupuncture in California.[29]

During the 1980s other states followed California's lead. Today there are more than ten thousand acupuncturists in the United States as well as three thousand medical doctors who perform acupuncture. Even though your health insurance may be more willing to pay for acupuncture performed by a medical doctor, my experience has demonstrated that a TCM practitioner who has devoted extensive study to the field of TCM has the background and training to treat you most effectively with acupuncture. The best way to find a good acupuncturist is to talk to people with your symptoms about their experiences with acupuncturists. If you are unable to find people in your area who can refer you, try contacting the National Certification Commission for Acupuncture and Oriental Medicine at (202) 232–1404. Their Web site is www.nccaom.org. Be sure to interview TCM practitioners before you begin treatment. Find out where they trained and for how long. Ask how long they have practiced and whether they have had experience treating your particular condition. This initial screening will help you find a good TCM practitioner who can help you.

11

Mind–Body Therapies

Modern medicine ... should use the overlooked resources of the mind and human spirit, which are the source of the inner forces of healing.
David McClelland, Ph.D., Harvard psychologist

During the long years of my search for alternative approaches that could help heal my lupus, I discovered six therapies that held promise for alleviating some of the psychological/neurologic symptoms I was experiencing. There is evidence that many of us with autoimmune illness have hyperactive sympathetic nervous systems. Involving our minds in relaxation exercises can reduce muscle tension, which in turn diminishes sympathetic nervous system activity. These integrated mind–body activities increase and balance energy on a cellular level, thus providing us with a better chance of getting well. Although I did not experience immediate results from any of these therapies, I have found that they have been a great help to me over an extended period of time.

Music

For many of us with chronic illness, listening to, singing, or playing music can be a nourishing and healing activity. Music affects us deeply on both a physical and emotional level. If carefully chosen, music can energize us, help us focus and process information, lower our pain level, make us feel less frustrated about our physical limitations, take our minds off our worries, and even assuage the loneliness that can accompany chronic illness. On a deeper level, music can help us believe that there is hope for us, that our lives are not over, that there is a reason for us to go on living.

Although research on the curative potential of music is quite new in the United States, many older cultures recognize the importance of music for healing. The Tibetan culture, for example, seems to have known for hundreds of years that music has medicinal effects. Tibetans believe that very low, sustained tones send out vibrational impulses that affect the body positively. These low notes may embrace human cells in a gentle vibrational "bath" that allows living cells to repel invaders and rejuvenate.

I experienced the effects of this music therapy when I attended a performance of Tibetan monks from the Drepung Loseling Monastery, who blow the long copper or brass horns called *dung chen* and chant in very low tones. The vocal chanting is sometimes done multiphonically, which means that a solitary singer simultaneously intones the three notes of a chord. These Tibetan singers achieve this ability only after many years of training. Following the performance, I slipped into the deepest slumber of my illness and felt calmer for a number of days. Tibetans traditionally take their elderly and ill people to hear these musical performances to encourage healing.

In hospitals in India, traditional Indian music is used to help people with hypertension and various forms of mental illness. The Chinese listen to music with such titles as "Liver" or "Bladder." They take these musical prescriptions just as they take herbal remedies. The roots of healing music probably date far back, past shamanic healing to the original bone flute playing forty-three thousand to eighty-two thousand years ago, and possibly before our species could talk, when we communicated through song or tone.[1]

Many of us are aware of our mood changes when we listen to music, but it has been only in the past decade or two that music has come to be considered a form of health therapy. Some hospitals encourage musicians to play or sing for critically ill patients to help soothe them, lowering their pain and anxiety levels. Many psychologists today also have special music playing in their clinics. Even creative visualization tapes often feature healing music in the background.

There is evidence that the right music can open our minds to new possibilities. It moves us beyond the left brain, which may keep us stuck on details, into the right brain, the more intuitive side. This allows us to gain access to the subconscious, the source of creativity and possibly happiness. Many of us with lupus can feel better integrating music into our days. Baroque lute music can instill calm, Mozart can perk us up intellectually, and the songs of Aretha Franklin can energize us physically. The important thing is to experience music that aids healing and at the same time keeps us alert and connected to the world around us.

Tai Chi

I was engaged in tai chi chuan (simply, "tai chi") some years before I became ill. An ancient form of martial art, tai chi is much "softer" than jujitsu, aikido, or karate. I chose the yang style, or the short form, from the many tai chi styles practiced today. A primary concept in tai chi is that of letting negative energy flow around or over you. One doesn't expend one's own precious energy trying to block negative energy. In fact, it is even possible to help negative energy move past you. This is a subtle concept, one that I didn't grasp too easily at first. But as I worked with my energy and the energies of the other people in the class, I began to feel more rooted, more stable, and more firmly planted and therefore started to feel as though I could let the negative energy around me flow over me. It helped me cope with a stressful job. I also noticed that I was walking the deck of our sailboat more securely; my balance was so much better that I stopped worrying about falling overboard.

I practice tai chi because I believe that it is a superior form of exercise.

Since the movements are slow, it takes control and strength in the body to perform the sequences. The movements may seem unusual to those of us who aren't used to disciplined body movement. Bending at the knees ever so slightly, with the back very straight, we imagine a rope or a ribbon coming out of the top of our heads, reaching up through the sky, connecting us to the universe. We also imagine ourselves "planted" in the earth, as though we have roots stretching down to the core of the planet. Once we're connected firmly through our feet and heads, we can proceed to learn the movements.

The intent of tai chi is to encourage the flow of the chi, or life spirit. So that we wouldn't create any blockages to the energy flow, my husband and I learned not to bend our wrists, because that blocks the flow of chi. We particularly loved practicing tai chi with a group. Meeting outdoors on summer evenings, we moved through the whole form together, gathering lots of spectators on the college square. As we learned the tai chi movement sequence over many weeks, some of us commented that we felt calmer and more content, and we became a circle of slow dancers reaching in unison for the positive energy around us.

Our American female tai chi teacher was quite demanding, moving around our circle, checking our postures, giving us individualized instruction. But when we were visited by a male instructor from Taiwan, we learned the nature of Asian tai chi discipline. He strutted around us, barking out corrections and even swatting us on our rears. Experiencing this teacher's approach taught me that the Chinese practice tai chi as a mental discipline as well as a physical one.

By focusing so carefully on the tai chi movements, I have learned to be conscious in the moment. I have become calmer and more willing to try to approach many things in my life through tai chi. Today I am often able to let much negative energy flow over, around, or through me. When we learn to think of energy in this way, we can meet problems much more effectively, knowing that we need to just let them flow, that we don't need to solve every problem that comes at us.

Once I became ill, I could not practice tai chi any longer. During those early years of my illness, I decided to perform tai chi in my mind, calling it *inner tai chi.* I imagined myself moving with our group through the sequences. Merely visualizing this helped me feel calm and even somewhat exercised, though I wasn't actually doing the movements. This is more proof to me of the important role the mind plays in healing.

Some years later, when I was strong enough and had lost at least some of the dizziness, I took up tai chi again. At first, all I could do was stand on my porch and perform the first hand movement sequences. Then I started bending a bit at the knee and sustaining that hold, which would cause me to be shaky afterward. But I kept at it and little by little was able to perform at an increasing pace. When I could finally manage the first third of the form with my husband coaching me if I faltered, I knew I wanted to study with an instructor again. By that time, I felt able to sink and turn with grace and strength, knowing that I wouldn't fall down from exhaustion.

Tai chi is too strenuous for those of us with severe lupus, but it can be a helpful exercise for the lupus patient with a mild to moderate form of the disease, even if you just stand or sit in one place and perform the arm movements. Video instructions are available, but I would recommend that you find a qualified tai chi teacher with whom to study. Explain your illness and ask whether the instructor can accommodate you. Even if you learn only the first third of the yang short form, you will have a helpful exercise sequence to perform each day. If you are not well enough to manage this, wait until you are feeling stronger.

WELLNESS BREATHING

As a lupus patient, I have found breathing exercises to be of great value. I have more energy, and I'm calmer and intellectually more focused since I began daily breathing exercises. During the darkest years of my illness I was extremely nervous and had difficulty relaxing. I became interested in meditating in an effort to calm my anxiety. I had to learn proper breathing techniques for meditation and also because I wanted to alleviate my panic attacks. The doctors told me that I was breathing too shallowly and that if I breathed more deeply and slowly, I could correct the oxygen/carbon dioxide imbalance in my system. When the carbon dioxide levels in the body fall from too rapid exhalation, the acid/alkaline balance in the blood is thrown off, which can provoke a panic attack. With this in mind, I decided to look for information on conscious breathing before I began to practice it.

At that time, my search turned up very little devoted to the subject of breathing but recognition of the importance of breathing, has been around for a long time. A number of ancient cultures acknowledge the spiritual aspects of breathing. The ancient Vedic (Hindu) mystics, for example, identified breath as the evidence of spirit in the body. In many languages the words for spirit and breath are the same: Sanskrit, *prana*; Greek, *pneume*; Hebrew, *ruack*; Latin, *spiritus*. As Andrew Weil states:

> Breath is nonmaterial, or at least, it straddles the border between material and nonmaterial reality. It . . . is the source of life and vitality. If breath is the movement of spirit in the body—a central mystery that connects us to all creation—then working with breath is a form of spiritual practice. It is also one that impacts health and healing, because how we breath both reflects the state of the nervous system and influences the state of the nervous system."[2]

When we are breathing correctly we will feel it as chi—a warm tingling in our hands and feet. This kind of breathing can treat many chronic conditions successfully. Our cells need oxygen. When they are underoxygenated, they cannot fight off invaders as they can when they have enough oxygen. By learning to breathe correctly, we can improve the circulation, blood pressure, heart rate, and digestion. We must learn to change the rhythm and depth of our breathing consciously. We can start simply by focusing our attention on our breath. Here are simple breathing exercises you can perform at home to improve your sense of well-being.

Put your tongue on the roof of your mouth and exhale your breath. Take breath in to a count of four, being sure to expand your rib cage and your diaphragm. If you have trouble doing this, lie on the floor. When you lie down, your breathing is the way it should be. Sit up and try to replicate that breathing. After taking your breath in to a count of four, hold your breath to a count of seven and release it slowly to a count of eight. Repeat this sequence eight times. Do the set of eight breaths twice a day.[3]

In his book *Conscious Breathing*, Gay Hendricks, Ph.D., gives us directions for a ten-minute daily breathing program that he suggests each of us should do every morning of our lives. The goal is to give ourselves a deep sense of centeredness. Hendricks says that hundreds of his students have reported a good supply of energy throughout the day, deeper and more restful sleep, disappearance of pain and tension, clearer concentration, greater calm, and easing of menstrual difficulties when they faithfully practice this breathing routine. This routine is more complicated than the previous one, but you will be glad you have taken the time to learn it and practice it.

1. Begin by lying on your back with your arms at your sides, knees bent, feet flat on the floor. Breathe deeply and slowly, in and out, arching the small of your back gently, and then flattening it against the floor on the outbreath. Move gently and slowly for two minutes. Then stretch our your legs and rest for a moment.

2. Still lying on your back, bring your legs up so that your feet are flat on the floor. Stretch your arms out in a T formation. Move one arm up the floor as the other moves down. Roll them slowly back and forth. Let your knees drop over toward the side where your arm is rolling down. Turn your head in the direction opposite your knees. Once you have mastered these coordinated movements, add your breathing. Breathe in and expand your belly as your knees near the floor, and then breathe out as your knees lift toward the midpoint. Begin another inbreath as your knees drop to the other side. Do the movements and the breathing very slowly, focusing on your sensations. Practice for two minutes. Then stretch out and rest for a few moments.

3. Sit upright. Using your nondominant hand, place your thumb on one nostril and your middle finger on the other. Breathe

slowly out one nostril and back in the same nostril. Close that
nostril and breathe out and in the other nostril. Switch only
after the inbreath. You should alternate these breaths for five
minutes. Your breathing may slow down, which is fine. Just let
it flow as it needs to. Continue for five minutes.[4]

I perform breathing exercises when I wake up and just before falling
asleep. I've also found that my daily walks in the woods are conducive to
practicing deep breathing. Out in nature, we are breathing oxygen that the
trees and other vegetation provide. This is one reason we need to preserve
our forests. The irony of deep breathing is that even though we need to do
it for our health, it may put us at risk, because the air we are breathing is
generally of increasingly poor quality. All of us who practice deep breathing should also be working to support clean air policy in our communities.

HYPNOSIS

One of my primary reasons for wanting to work with hypnosis was to find
a way to encourage my subconscious mind to calm my body and minimize
my lupus symptoms. I wanted to ask my body to recover its healthy state.
At this time I was deeply ill. No matter how much I rested, I felt exhausted
virtually all the time. I also had constant pain in my neck, head, and upper
back as well as my wrists, hands, ankles, and feet. My eyes were sensitive to
light, and I had difficulty reading. My ears rang much of the time. I was
always dizzy and often needed to grasp walls or furniture for support.
There seemed to be no relief from these symptoms; they were with me
when I went to bed and when I awoke.

After a fairly long search, I found a counselor with a doctorate who was
trained in Ericksonian hypnosis and was willing to work with me at home.
During our first meeting, we talked about how we might encourage my
immune system to normalize again after so many years of hyperactivity.
The hypnotherapist offered a number of creative approaches that he
thought might help.

Each week at our appointment he asked me to close my eyes, take deep breaths, and relax each part of my body. This moved me into a trancelike state. Once I was in a trance, we thanked my immune system for helping defend my body against illness. We then addressed my T cells, thanking them specifically for all the work they had done on my behalf. During this time I began to imagine my T cells as busy little creatures who needed a rest. I told them they were continuing to work too hard when there was no need for it. Wouldn't they like to take a holiday? I suggested that my T cells relax, lie in the sun, read the paper, drink a margarita, take the dog for a walk, get a massage. Although I found this amusing on one level, on another level, I believe that by thanking my T cells and asking them to change their behavior, I encouraged them to calm down and stop attacking my own body.

While I was under trance, the hypnotherapist also suggested that I find the truths I needed to know at that time. The psychiatrist Milton H. Erickson believed that we each carry all our truths within us and that the challenge is for us to get in touch with those truths. I finally was able to face the truth that I was terrified of dying. I was still young, had enjoyed an interesting life, and had brought a certain exuberance to living. I felt that I had made some contributions to society and wanted to go on assisting in some way. For that, I needed not only to live but also to get well enough to function again.

Another truth I began to confront was that I had grown to hate my body; it had become such a burden that I could barely drag it around with me. I was also full of self-doubt, thinking that I may have brought on my lupus but not knowing what I had done to cause it. In my worst moments, I lapsed into wondering why a higher power would be punishing me. It also appeared to me that some of my caretakers were disgusted with me for being so ill and therefore so "difficult." Then, too, I was terrified of becoming a vegetable, a person who would always have to be cared for by other people.

As I began to look at these frightening and painful truths under the guidance of the hypnotherapist, I gradually seemed to find ways of bringing my own creativity to resolving each issue. Even when I was out of trance, ideas began to appear to me for dealing with the particular challenges I was facing. The hypnotherapist also skillfully validated my "new self," who was beginning to emerge from the illness. When I was angry, he validated the anger. When I was sad, he validated the sadness. Since I had a long history of difficulty in working with conventional medical doctors, he helped me design approaches that assisted me in dealing with doctors who are poor communicators. The hypnotherapist often said that, "being listened to unconditionally is necessary for our good health." It's true that we all need to feel that we have importance in the world. In a highly competitive, materialistic culture like ours, where the sick are often avoided and made to feel unwanted and unloved, those of us who are chronically ill can feel validated if someone simply listens to us.

The hypnotherapist's work with me in trance led me to an understanding that even though I had not been taught as a child to listen to my inner needs, I could now learn to take care of myself. Indeed, it was critical that I take control and actually manage my own recovery. Under hypnosis I began to feel secure in the knowledge that I had the inner resources to find and use many approaches for healing. Ultimately, I began to believe that I truly was in control of my own healing.

Although I have no conscious recollection of trying to think of what to do next to feel better, under hypnosis, my subconscious was apparently doing a lot of work for me. I knew this because I often heard myself say something that startled me, and I'd find myself asking, "Was it me who just said that? Where did that come from?" In some ways, I felt as though I were finding a new personality with which I needed to get acquainted. This was intriguing. Was it possible that as a result of hypnosis, I was taking on a stronger persona that would help me when I recovered from lupus? Was there beginning to be a break in my illness that would allow me to contemplate a future? Many of the problems brought on by lupus began to recede into the background. As the physical symptoms, fears, anger, and confusion provoked by my illness dissipated, I began to see myself again as a healthy, thriving, loving, and loved human being.

Because I felt that my sessions under hypnosis were alleviating my lupus symptoms and helping me live with the complexities of being chronically ill,

I searched for research that might validate what I was experiencing. I found only one study that reported the successful use of hypnosis for a patient with SLE. I describe this study in some detail, because it shows how important hypnosis can be as a therapy for SLE. In this study, a forty-one-year-old registered nurse with SLE went to the therapist hoping to find relief from her severe pain and dependence on medications. She said that the medications were affecting her ability to do her work and maintain her social life. In the first session the therapist taught her deep muscle relaxation techniques, to which she responded positively. She stated that she had a "wonderful feeling of floating and freedom," adding that it "relaxed me, even at such a high point of physical pain and mental anxiety."[5]

During the second session her use of the feelings of lightness and floating, cooling, and counting upward helped deepen her trance state. The therapist taped the session, during which she experienced becoming lighter and lighter until she was floating on a cloud. The patient listened to the tape twice a day for the following week and reported that it helped. In subsequent sessions she was taught to minimize her pain with a dissociation technique. She felt herself "flying away from the pain" and "soaring" into a time and place where she had no pain. Words the therapist used were "blue sky," "gentle and cool breeze," "freshness of air," and "sound of birds." This helped her gain distance from her pain.

Systematic desensitization—encouraging a patient to approach the situation and be less sensitive to it—helped ease her fear and panic in trying to work with an ophthalmologist who had administered a laser beam treatment, which may have caused blindness in her left eye. This patient also learned how to reinterpret pain signals to trigger pleasurable sensations. The therapist suggested that she imagine wearing gloves to protect her hands while she pressed a handful of cold snow to her head to relieve her severe headaches. She then could picture the cold of the snow numbing her head. This worked so well that she was able to discontinue all pain medication while continuing to taper off her dosages of Valium and sedatives.

In another session, the therapist hypnotized her and suggested that she would no longer need to take sleeping medication but instead could rely on herself, nature, and relaxation. He also told her that her faith and self-confidence would be more helpful to her than artificial sleep aids. This allowed her, over the next week, to discontinue the use of her sleeping medication. In the course of these sessions this nurse with lupus became quite competent at using autohypnosis to help herself cope with anxiety, pain, and sleep problems. In the therapist's view this was a highly successful application of hypnosis for an SLE patient. Not only did this treatment help control her pain, but she also gained self-esteem, confidence, and a sense of self-control and general zest for living.

Hypnosis can have positive benefits for lupus patients. To find a licensed, academically qualified hypnotherapist, call your state licensing agency for a list of these professionals in your area. Then carefully interview them, looking for a hypnotherapist who has worked with chronically ill people. Be sure to interview some of his or her clients by telephone before you make a choice. Try to work with a hypnotherapist whose fees your health plan will reimburse.

Neurolinguistic Programming

Neurolinguistic programming (NLP) is a form of hypnosis that I have used to curb my anxiety. These simple, but powerful exercises have helped me manage to be in crowds and ride in cars and planes again. Even more exciting is the power of NLP to help patients moderate their autoimmune response. This is groundbreaking research. Studies documenting changes in immunoglobulin levels by the use of visual imagery are rare. As of early 1996, William L. Mundy, M.D., knew of only one such study. Dr. Mundy, a psychiatrist, believes that specific emotions produce chemical changes in the body. We all have emotions, which, in Mundy's opinion, are tools to help us respond to the world. According to Mundy, it is the inappropriate use of feelings when responding to stressors, not chemicals, that causes our problems.

Dr. Mundy thinks allergens are harmless unless the mind and body get the idea that they should be considered "enemies." Why do the mind and body decide that they're enemies? Stress seems to be the trigger. It may be the stress of a bacteria or virus, but it also can be a stress-producing emotion. In trying to protect us, the immune cells go on the attack. That immune cell response can make us sick with allergies. It also can make us sick by attacking our own tissue, as in autoimmune disease. An allergy could be thought of as a phobia.

How can we change the actions of our immune cells? A simple NLP technique originally meant to cure phobias may help stop our overreaction and the unnecessary response of our immune cells. Dr. Mundy has had success using the following exercise to treat patients with autoimmune conditions.

1. The patient is asked to name the allergens and describe her symptoms as the allergy attack occurs.
2. The patient then is asked to think of a product like the allergic substance but which causes no symptoms. For example, you could drink coconut milk, even though you have severe allergies to dairy products.
3. The patient then is asked to imagine herself looking at herself across the room, through a thick Plexiglas shield, and seeing herself eating the product that is healthy.
4. With this image in mind, the patient is encouraged to be aware that her immune system *knows* that food is healthy.
5. The patient then is asked to see herself eating the allergic food while bearing in mind that her immune system knows that food is perfectly healthy and acceptable.
6. The patient has been watching herself eating both kinds of food and keeping the healthy image in mind.
7. She now comes back from across the room and sits where she is seated. This integrates her immune system, focusing the knowledge that it no longer needs to act mistakenly, as it did in the past. The patient is contacting her immune response on a cellular level in this way, but she must remain open to the concept.

Dr. Mundy has seen good responses in a pediatric group using this approach. This technique is called *reframing*, perceiving oneself in a similar situation but with a different frame of reference. As Dr. Mundy says, "It is awesome that the mind/body is able to make sense of a metaphorical play, made up on the spot, and stop the immune cells from overreacting."[6] Mind seems to exist, he thinks, on a cellular level.

Mundy is attempting to use his modified imagery techniques on the devastating autoimmune diseases of multiple sclerosis, SLE, and rheumatoid arthritis. He believes that many of us with autoimmune illness have had early depression that was ignored, that went undiagnosed and untreated. He says that many kinds of imagery can work for us. For example, one of his patients with lupus visualized little versions of Puff the Magic Dragon carrying buckets of ice to her affected joints; in this way, she was able to eliminate 70 percent to 90 percent of her pain. Mundy does not think that we need to understand completely how the mind works, only that we need to be grateful that the mind does work so effectively for us.[7] You may benefit from working with an NLP practitioner who has used Mundy's exercise with autoimmune patients. Try networking in your city or town or checking the Yellow Pages for a person trained in NLP techniques. If you are unable to locate such a practitioner, you may want to ask a family member or friend to talk you carefully through Mundy's exercise each day.

BIOFEEDBACK

This form of mind—body therapy can be effective for those of us with stress-sensitive chronic illness. Biofeedback uses electrical instruments to monitor particular symptoms, such as muscle tension, brain wave activity, and pulse. These instruments then show us the activities they are monitoring. When we're hooked to the monitoring device, we can learn to modify the body's activities by listening to the tone of the sound the machine makes or by watching the light. This is a credible way for people to measure the level of relaxation they're attaining. Slowing the heart rate, regulating the flow of blood to various parts of the body, and even changing brain waves by responding to lights or sounds is all possible with biofeedback technology.

The psychologist Richard Surriet of Duke University Medical Center has used biofeedback to teach people with type II diabetes, an autoimmune disease, to raise the level of glucose tolerance in their bodies through biofeedback. Before biofeedback training, these diabetics did not require insulin, but they did have difficulty maintaining their blood glucose levels in the safety range even with a special diet.

In the 1980s researchers at the Stanford University Arthritis Center discovered that using relaxation exercises can help alleviate the stress and discomfort of rheumatoid arthritis. With some people, it appears that it even may increase the body's production of the natural painkillers called endorphins. Thus, relaxation techniques may produce an analgesic response. Research also has shown that biofeedback can help mitigate the pain and accompanying tension felt by patients with arthritis and allow them to sleep better. In another study, an arthritic group using biofeedback felt much better. An erythrocyte sedimentation rate blood test, measuring the activity of the disease, showed that the immune system had held stable against the disease or the arthritis actually had abated.[8]

PROGRESSIVE RELAXATION

This simple approach to body relaxation can be helpful in reducing stress levels. First, find a quiet place to sit. Beginning with your feet and lower legs, tense and relax the muscle groups in those parts of your body. Each muscle group is tensed for a slow count of ten seconds and then released for another ten seconds. Moving up your body, in order, tense and relax your upper legs, buttocks, stomach, and so on. Reaching your upper body, tense and relax both forearms, upper arms, forehead, both eyes, the nose, both cheeks, the mouth, and then the neck. It's important that you concentrate on the muscles as they unclench, taking a moment to appreciate the sensations that flow from them. This method is easy to learn and can be done anywhere, anytime, to lower your stress levels.

These self-soothing approaches can help calm us and, in doing so, can likewise calm our illness. We will benefit for the remainder of our lives by using music, tai chi, wellness breathing, hypnosis, biofeedback relaxation, and progressive relaxation to encourage the mind—body balance that is the basis of true health.

12

Caring for Your Spirit

May I be at peace.
May my heart remain open.
May I awaken to the light of my own true nature.
May I be healed.
May I be a source of healing for all beings.

Buddhist prayer

Learning to care for ourselves when we have lupus involves what I call "tending the spirit." Just as we tend our gardens, our families, and our careers, tending our psychological and emotional health is important for those of us who are chronically ill. When our minds and hearts are at peace, we have a greater chance of recovering our physical health. Even if we are unable to recover completely, tending our spirit can help us better cope with our illness over the long term.

Putting our minds at rest concerning the cause of our lupus is one of the healthiest ways to tend our spirits. A haunting question for many of us with this illness is whether we brought it on ourselves. Are we being punished, we ask ourselves, for something we have done? Whether we are religious or nonreligious, many of us wonder why we are being required to suffer so much. After struggling with this issue for many years, I finally concluded that illness is generally a random event. I think that we are not being singled out, nor do we bring these illnesses on ourselves, except perhaps in cases of substance abuse or poor personal health habits. Most of us must be careful not to blame ourselves for being ill. As we think back over the patterns of our lives, it may seem in retrospect that we were working too hard, perhaps carrying too much responsibility or too much stress, but we did not choose to bring lupus into our lives. It came upon us through a complex set of circumstances, many of which we could not have controlled.

In my own case, only when I stopped blaming myself or a higher power for causing my illness was I able to believe that I could recover from lupus. At that point, gentle, supportive words like *honor, empower, holistic,* and *cocreate* began to take on special meaning for me. I found that using these words helped me rewrite my story, changing the theme from one of illness to one of renewed health. Integrating these kinds of words into our vocabularies assists us in shifting our concentration away from the disease and toward the beneficial activities our bodies perform for us even when we are ill.

When illness comes into our lives, it can be instructive to reexamine our perspective on health. What is health? Does it mean the complete absence of pain? High energy? The physical ability to perform strenuous work? Is it only a physical definition? Does it have an emotional/psychological component as well? While we each may have our own definition of health, many of us have come to support a holistic meaning of the concept. In its totality, health seems to have to do with our thoughts and emotions as well as our physical stamina. In general, if we feel good about the world, about ourselves, and about other people, we're healthy.

Health need not even involve physical strength. Some people who are wheelchair-bound, for example, or physically disabled in other ways can be very healthy. They may have positive attitudes that allow them to perform well in the world even with a disability. Through the years of my lupus, I've met a number of people who seemed spiritually, psychologically, and emotionally healthy even though they were physically ill. On the other hand, we all know able-bodied people who are so damaged in terms of their emotional and psychological health that they function poorly in many aspects of their lives. Are they healthy? Most of us would agree that they are not.

By keeping our spirits intact and vibrant, we can be healthy even if we are physically limited by illness. Tending our spirits will help us rise above illness and move through its difficulties. In this chapter I offer a variety of suggestions, from my own experience, for nourishing our spirits while we are chronically ill.

HEALING THOUGHTS

Many of us grew up thinking that prayers were written by someone else and read from a book. When I became ill and in need of solace, we couldn't find many prayers that adequately spoke to my feeling of devastation and my need for reassurance. I decided to create my own spiritual practices. What should I say? I wondered. Did I need to appeal to a "higher power"? Did I need to quote from Scripture? After much pondering, I finally decided that spiritual practice could be anything that helped me reach the ultimate kindness that surrounds each of us. That decision freed me to range beyond spoken prayer. Testing the waters, I began singing my prayers, then whistled my prayers, then chanted my prayers. When I grew stronger, I bellowed my prayers, and, finally, I began to dance my prayers. Those prayers surprised me with their power. They hovered, dived, and swirled; they encircled and cushioned me on a carpet ride along the path to recovery. Early on, I prayed mostly for my own healing. Then I read about the Vietnamese Buddhist Thich Nhat Hanh walking his meditation, striding slowly and purposefully in his bare feet, praying for peace in the world, kissing the ground in humility. Shortly thereafter, on my halting daily walks, I began to envision happiness for all living beings, believing that my simple prayers might resonate enough to help someone else.

Is there any proof that what we do with our minds can affect other people in a positive way? In fact, research that the Russians and others have been conducting suggests the incredible power of our minds to reach other people. In one study, Russian technicians put people in lead-lined boxes and asked other people thousands of miles away to send them mental messages. The "lead-lined recipients" had no idea what sorts of messages were coming or even whether any messages were being sent. Amazingly, they received most of the messages. Sometimes these were spoken messages; sometimes they were only mental images. In either case, human extrasensory perception seems to be very much at work here.[1]

There is also evidence from pure science that our minds are interconnected. Dr. John Bell, an Irish physicist, discovered in 1964 that once two objects touch, or are even momentarily physically close, they will always have an affinity for each other, no matter where they go in the universe. If something affects one of the objects, it will always affect the other object as well. This concept is called the *Bell theorem*.[2] An exciting idea, it has direct application to prayer. If someone we met when we were five years old, for example, and whom we have not seen since, prays for us, according to the Bell theorem, we could respond positively. This is "New Physics" at its best—the idea that even though energy appears chaotic, inside the chaos are intertwined patterns of stability, compatibility, and connectedness.

Can we bring about healing through our spiritual practices? The answer appears to be yes. Building on the ideas from Russian research and New Physics, fascinating studies done on bacteria, yeast, and fungi growth have shown that people can use their minds to stop the growth of these pathogens and the diseases they cause. Larry Dossey, M.D., says, "It seems that ordinary people have the ability to bring about biological changes in other living organisms. This suggests that everyone may possess innate healing abilities, at least to some degree."[3] Dr. Dossey goes on to state,

> More than 130 controlled laboratory studies show, in general, that prayer or a prayer-like state of compassion, empathy, and love can bring about healthful changes in many types of living things, from humans to bacteria. This does not mean prayer always works, any

more than drugs and surgery always work, but that statistically speaking, prayer is effective.[4]

Spiritual practice can calm us, but it also needs to spur us to be active rather than passive. Not only can we pray for ourselves and others in order to tend our spirits, but we also must *do* things for ourselves and others. Our innate compassion, our respect for people, our basic kindness can lead us to helping people and ourselves. In this way, we plant the seeds of miracles in the most ordinary daily activities. Instead of waiting for perfect health and happiness before we do anything, we can start using our daily spiritual practice, our good sense, our pragmatism, our courage, our tenacity, and our persistence for helping others. The continuing miracle is that we can all contribute, no matter how ill we may be.

Many of us wonder whether there is a specific form of prayer or spiritual practice that works best. Dossey reports that the research shows that it doesn't really matter what we say. We can intone a long, formal, healing prayer that will be heard. Or we can say simply, "Thy will be done." That will also be heard. We even can say, "Heal Marilyn." Or we can just think, without verbalizing, "Help John in his current situation." As we visualize John in his environment, he will be affected positively by our thoughts. Or we can dance slowly, holding the image of a healthy, happy John in our minds as we move. All of these approaches are valid for healing; they will all resonate through time, space, and matter. The important issue here is to make certain that we send only positive, healing thoughts. When we send these prayers and spiritual essences out, we are helping alter energy patterns for the better around the whole planet.

In order to develop your spiritual practice, try writing or speaking your own prayers and meditations. Then sing them, chant them, walk them, dance them. Send your spiritual thoughts out to people and other living things who need healing. This is an active way for you to help the world. Take comfort in the certainty that your prayers are having a positive effect wherever you send them. By engaging in healing thoughts, you are caring for your own spirit in a vibrant, nurturing way.

ALLEVIATING LONELINESS

Another way of tending our spirits is to deal with the loneliness that long-term illness may bring. When my unnamed illness struck me, I felt completely alone. No one I knew could understand my suffering, sealed as I was inside a shell of depression, pain, exhaustion, and confusion. In the course of many conversations with chronically ill people over the years, I've searched for ideas on how to ameliorate this deep loneliness. One piece of wisdom I learned from these discussions is that we must learn to be alone when we are ill and be strong enough not to call that loneliness. Personally, this has been a difficult adjustment for me, because I am by nature gregarious. But I found that as I became less frightened of my still undiagnosed illness, I was able to spend more time alone with my own thoughts.

Over time, the process of learning to assuage my loneliness involved relearning how to think about myself. Working with the hypnotherapist, I began to separate myself from the illness, so that I could get back in touch with myself. Putting the illness aside, I rediscovered my courage, intelligence, curiosity, and sense of humor, and realized that I had a very good friend in *me*. Although this may sound strange, I believe that many of us in Western society are estranged from ourselves; we're so busy, we take little time for the reflection we need to stay in touch with our true essence. As a lupus patient, you may find it beneficial to concentrate on mentally separating yourself from your illness. Remember that your illness is not you, and you are not your illness. Your illness is only one aspect of your life. If you blame yourself for being ill, changing your thinking in this way will lower your stress levels and help you enjoy your own company more, thereby lessening your loneliness.

In addition to becoming our own best friend, we may need to invite people to visit when we are ill. These days people can be so busy that they often feel they have little time for visiting. This is causing our social networks to collapse. Many of our friends and family visited in the first year or two of my illness, but by the third year we needed to start inviting them. People seemed to have low tolerance for long-term illness. On the other hand, many people who came to visit stayed too long, and I became exhausted. The "perfect visitor" arrived with a book to loan and stories to tell and stayed one hour. This was more than sufficient to keep me from feeling lonely.

To better tend our spirits, we need our visitors to bring stories of the outside world. After a year or two of relative isolation brought on by lupus, memories may begin to fade. In my own experience, I forgot what cross-country ski trails looked like because I couldn't get to them. I couldn't remember our city parks or what it was like to eat in a restaurant. I needed to hear descriptions of places and activities. Many visitors wove wonderful stories on their visits, and I was grateful for all the afternoons and evenings of stimulating conversation.

Staying connected to the outside world is important for monitoring health. There is evidence that lupus patients who are isolated and lonely at home may not take good care of themselves. Proper management of SLE requires regular assessment of symptoms, energy conservation, protection from sunlight, infection control, medication side-effect information, and fatigue management. In a special study, telephone calls from nurses were found to encourage lupus patients to take better care of themselves. The phone sessions were standardized to target six behaviors: self-care activities in managing fatigue, patient's communication skills, removing barriers to medical care, medication self-management, symptom monitoring, and stress-control methods. A goal of the phone counselors was to reinforce the lupus patients' assertiveness. The study found conclusively that telephone calls can be effective in improving lupus patients' ability to function. "Physical function and social support were significantly improved for SLE patients who received this specific telephone support. The patient's management of fatigue also improved. The phone consultations also appeared to have a positive [effect] on the level of arthritis pain reported by the participants."[3]

Other activities that can help us feel less lonely when we're ill include helping our children or neighbor children with their schoolwork, playing with and caring for pets, attending religious or spiritual services, telephoning other people who are ill to give them encouragement, participating in lupus support groups, and writing or E-mailing friends to stay in touch. If you are homebound by your lupus, ask yourself whether you have enough visitors to keep you connected with the world. Are they sharing the stories you need to hear to help nurture and support your spirit? Do visitations amplify your fatigue? If so, how can you manage to become less fatigued when people visit? If you need more visitors, how can you encourage them? Are you able to stay in touch, at least by phone, with health professionals for monitoring your self-care? Addressing each of these issues will help you care for your spirit in a healthy and productive way.

COMFORTING ACTIVITIES

There are many activities that can bring us interesting hours when we're ill. Although we may not be able to manage much stimulation, it is important for us to keep our minds active. Setting up creative atmospheres for ourselves helps us stay in touch with our abilities and plans for the future. Libraries can be a great source of help. The "Books for the Blind and Disabled" service, available through your public library, offers an array of fiction and nonfiction to those of us debilitated by illness. When you apply for the program, you will receive a special tape player on permanent loan and catalogues from which you can borrow books on tape. This program has provided me with countless hours of interesting narration and dialogue. Another service that can assist you is the National Library Service for the Blind and Physically Handicapped. You can also register with them and receive books on tape through the mail. See the resource section of this book for the address and phone number of this organization.

Writing activities can assist us in feeling better when we are chronically ill. Keeping a daily journal may help us rise above our symptoms and gain the awareness that we have a life beyond illness. Writing letters helps us stay in touch with friends and family. The creative activity of writing poetry, articles, and short stories stimulates our minds. I was fortunate to be able to continue my newsletter writing/editing business for the first two years of my illness. Working part-time at home, if we're able, keeps us involved and brings in an income that can help cover our health care costs.

In addition to mental activities, physical exertion also helps tend our spirits. When I could finally walk steadily, I started playing ball with a neighbor's puppy. Then I began walking the puppy around our yard, eventually making four laps around the periphery of our acre each day. If you are able, try walking a quarter of a mile, even if you do it very slowly. You may be surprised at your body's ability to carry you that distance. Keep at it every day, being careful not to overextend yourself. Your body and mind need this physical activity to regain a healthy balance.

Gardening is an excellent activity to take our minds off our illness. Even if we can only sit in a chair and talk to the person who is tending the garden, it gets us involved with nurturing living things. When we're rewarded with colorful flowers and tasty, organic vegetables, the work seems well worth it. If you want to garden but are too weak to bend or kneel, try other positions. The husband of an acquaintance of mine built her raised, waist-high vegetable beds so that she could garden without bending or stooping. During a period of debilitating illness, the mother of a friend lay on her stomach on a mat in order to weed and harvest her beloved strawberries.

Caring for a pet also can bring us great comfort when we are ill. A new body of research verifies that pets can help the healing process significantly. At least one study has shown that the presence of pets is more therapeutic than the presence of family members. Perhaps that is because pets are unconditional in the love they extend to us. When I became ill, we had only one cat, but over time a number of abandoned pets found their way to our door until we had six cats and a dog. They were a great comfort to me, and caring for them helped me step back from my illness and be concerned for other creatures. Spending many hours in bed each day, time passed more quickly and sleep came more easily with two or three cats snuggled up to me.

Some of us who are physically challenged by lupus can be aided by specially trained dogs that assist the physically disabled. These dogs possess the intelligence, problem-solving abilities, even temperaments, and desire to please people that is necessary to help physically challenged people. Studies have shown that people with disabilities who have service dogs score higher in terms of self-esteem and psychological well-being. Trained service animals also moderate stress, improve motivation, decrease serum cholesterol, and diminish loneliness. For more information on finding one of these dogs to join your family and become your pet/companion, see the resource section at the end of this book. My pets' companionship has helped me recover from lupus. If you don't already have a pet, consider getting one. It will reward you with countless hours of entertainment and affection. Rather than buying a dog or cat at a pet store, consider adopting an abandoned pet that needs a home. Visit your local animal shelter and bring home a dog or cat that otherwise might be destroyed.

Art projects can bring comfort and stimulation during illness. Some of us may have wanted to tap our artistic sides but never had the opportunity. Using the creative side of the brain can calm us when we are ill. If you have a developed ability at art, be sure to continue with that activity. If you are a beginner, as I was, get a copy of *Drawing on the Right Side of the Brain,* by Betty Edwards; find a pencil and sketch pad; and begin her exercises. Practice every day. You may even want to find an instructor. I've found that I enjoy drawing and have moved on to using pastels and watercolors. To find the artist in you, ask yourself what you always have wanted to do that's creative? Buy instructional books or borrow them from the library, find someone to teach you, and make a start at becoming an artist or a craftsperson. These activities will help you care for your spirit in an enjoyable, positive way.

HAVING COMPASSION FOR OURSELVES AND OTHERS

During the early years of my illness, I needed tenderness and encouragement but found very little of it beyond my family and friends. There is a curious tendency in this society to blame people who are sick. What is prompting this lack of compassion toward people who are suffering from illness? One explanation appears in the book *Between Heaven and Earth: A Guide to Chinese Medicine.* In it the authors say, "Western either-or thinking prompts us to conceive of illness within a narrow logic that fails us by its lack of breadth. We blame the victim by asserting that people cause their own sickness; hence, with a positive attitude, they can make themselves well. So, if they don't get well, it's their own fault."[6]

This societal blaming may be one of the reasons why it's difficult to find words of encouragement when we are ill. Often we don't even get encouragement from our own conventional Western doctors. In fact, some of them may discourage us actively from daring to believe that we can recover from chronic illness. I've had conventional doctors tell me that they didn't want to give me false hope for recovery. One day I was discussing this issue with a friend of who had recovered from serious illness. Her advice was that in light of the lack of compassion in our culture, we each need to focus on being our own best source of inspiration. "Be your own cheer-leader," she said.

Many of the world's major religions deal with suffering and the necessity of helping those who are afflicted. Buddhism, for example, teaches very clearly that we all suffer, that we must be aware of the suffering each of us experiences, and that we need to have compassion for ourselves and others. If we translate these ideas to our own illness, we may be able to diminish the effects of our suffering by having more compassion for ourselves. When we are so ill that we are unable to read a page and understand it, we need to accept that and not blame ourselves. Meanwhile, comforting ourselves with activities at which we can succeed—like brushing the dog, painting a flower with watercolors, making a salad, or writing a letter—will help us maintain compassion for ourselves. If we don't have the energy to kneel in the garden and weed for more than fifteen minutes, rather than becoming frustrated and angry with ourselves, we would do better to feel gratitude that we can work even that long.

To help us develop more compassion for ourselves, we can write affir-mations each day. An affirmation is a short positive statement about a way to think or a goal we want to achieve. The key to effective affirmations is to write them as though they have been accomplished. "I am well," "I am happy," "I am no longer nervous," "My gardens are flourishing," "I am walk-ing ten miles a week"—these are a few examples. We must write each of these sentences ten times to allow for our subconscious to absorb the infor-mation. I started this activity when I was very ill. Some days I could barely write twenty sentences. Today I still write hundreds of positive, creative affirmations each week on all sorts of subjects—primarily the hope I have for a healthier, more productive life. This exercise helped me enormously at sustaining the belief that I could recover my health.

Those near us may demonstrate their compassion for us in gentle, deeply touching ways. When I was a thousand days into the illness, wondering whether I would survive it, my husband did a lovely thing for me. He said that he had been giving a great deal of thought to the fact that while athletes and scholars get medals and degrees, sick people never gain recognition for the Olympic task of enduring a debilitating illness. To correct what he thought was an oversight, he staged a ceremony in which he portrayed me as a hero, someone who was going the long distance, who was not giving up, who deserved a hearty congratulations for her ability to endure. Then he presented me with an engraved gold medal hanging on a red, white, and blue ribbon. The inscription read, "To Sharon. After 1,000 days of illness, still an inspiration to us all."

Although those of us with lupus may be able to manage only small, quiet accomplishments, we must focus on our successes in order to keep believing that we will recover. Enduring difficulty and searching creatively for solutions is the very essence of heroism. Each one of us is, in fact, a hero. As you care for your spirit, ask yourself whether you regard yourself as a hero. If you don't, concentrate on how you might change your thinking to see yourself more as a hero. Each time you accomplish something that's been difficult for you, give yourself a "medal," perhaps in the form of a gourmet meal, a massage, or a floral bouquet, and quietly reflect on your heroism.

As lupus patients, we can benefit by remembering that we are doing the best we can. We will make progress every day, and we will have many setbacks. It is important to have compassion for ourselves and other people, because it nourishes the spirit. If we nurture ourselves, we will feel better, heal faster, and be more content with ourselves and the people around us. Ask yourself whether you are being compassionate enough with yourself during this time of illness. Do you rest? Do you eat well? Are you honest with people about how your illness limits you? Do you ask for help when you need it? Are you compassionate with other people? Are you a good listener for those who need your friendship and counsel? Attention to these spiritual issues will help you heal yourself and deepen your love for those around you.

Another serious problem for those of us struck down by illness has to do with how we can continue to think of ourselves as important to the world when we become so incapacitated. In a culture obsessed with being productive, how do we adjust to the guilt, frustration, anger, and even fear we feel when we no longer can produce? This is the same dilemma many people experience when they retire. We Americans tend to define ourselves by our jobs. In the past this was primarily a problem for men, but now it applies equally to women. With the impact of feminism over the past thirty years, many women today define themselves through their work: "I am a teacher." "I am a stockbroker." "I am a carpenter." "I am a tug- boat captain." When we become ill with chronic disease, we may be in dan- ger of losing our sense of self. No longer able to perform paying work, we may feel anxious and depressed at being unable to make our contribution to society any longer.

When I was confronted by this dilemma, I found encouragement from three Christian women who were visiting to say healing prayers for me. I had been telling them how heartsick I was at being so useless. They argued that I was a living being and through that fact alone I had value. Even though I might not be making an obvious contribution, they said, I should realize that I was contributing in another way—by giving others an oppor- tunity for personal growth through their service to me.

More help with my sense of self came from a Tibetan Buddhist who visited our home. I was telling him how exhausted I was from listening to people's problems when they visited. He observed that many people in America seem to be alone, with no one to confide in. I wanted a way to begin contributing again, he said, and here it was. I could be a confidante to people who simply needed someone to listen. This gentle Tibetan talked at length about how we must move into people's sorrow in order to have compassion for them. Compassion is the key. That is what we can give the world through our spiritual practice and our actions. Although this idea is not prominent in our materialistic culture, he said, by feeling more compassion, expressing more "loving kindness," we can become happier people.

Buddhist thought also has taught me that while we may not be able to change a circumstance, we can change the way we think about it. If you feel unnecessary in the world now because you have a chronic illness, explore the following questions about yourself, searching for a way to change your thinking, enhance your self-esteem, and care for your spirit while you continue to live with lupus. Do you feel less important now that you have lupus? Can you analyze why you feel that way? What is contributing to your ruptured sense of self? Write down all your ideas. How can you begin to change your perspective? Who can you talk to about this? What can you read that can help you feel loved and important again, even though you are ill? Every day, write three positive affirmations, ten times each, that can help you change the way you think about yourself while you are ill—for example, "I am loved, and I am love" or "I am valuable as I am."

AVOIDING MEDIA VIOLENCE

One of the best ways to care for the spirit is to avoid the portrayal of violence wherever we find it. I had been boycotting media violence for years, even before I became ill, because I am convinced that it is a dangerous influence. A steady diet of violence is one of the factors contributing to the demise of our society. Numerous studies indicate that media violence has a hand in the proliferation of weapons in our culture. As people become more afraid of weaponry, they trust each other less. As violence spreads, therefore, it is destroying our sense of community, the very fabric of our democratic country.

Many of us with lupus have nervous system symptoms, as I did, which can take the form of depression, anxiety, even paranoia. When I became ill, violence on television, in films, and in the newspapers shocked and upset me. I began strictly avoiding all forms of this violence, which helped me feel more hopeful. Without any violence coming across the airwaves in our home, my husband noticed that he, too, felt better psychologically.

In his book *Spontaneous Healing,* Andrew Weil encourages us to "try a one day news fast. Do not read, watch, or listen to any news for a day and see how you feel. Then, try to do two days of news fasting the following week. Then extend your news fast to three days."[7] Continue this trend until you listen to very little news. If you feel that you must keep up with what's going on in the world, read only the sections of the newspaper that do not dwell on violence. Do not watch television news. By avoiding violence in the media, you will guard your spirit from being tainted by the cynicism and fear that permeates our violent culture. This will lower your stress levels and consequently may help heal your nervous system symptoms.

HEALING IN NATURE

One aspect of my life that strongly influenced my healing was living on a one-acre property in a rural area. The relative peace of the place provided a low-stress environment, allowing me to relax as much as the illness would allow. We've since moved to another property that has even more native vegetation. Here on Wild Goose Hill, the trees attract wildlife in many forms. Flocks of birds pass through, fueling up at our bird feeders. On the ground rest decaying trunks that provide refuge for many small creatures, such as chipmunks, squirrels, moles, mice, and even bats, which eat the mosquitoes breeding in our pond. Black-tailed deer pass through, and raccoons snack at our compost pile. We occasionally see a coyote and often hear them yipping in the darkness. Once we saw a black bear eating wild blackberries near our home.

With the passing of the seasons, creating bouquets from brilliant rhododendrons in spring, then colorful dahlias in late August, and finally September-blooming asters, I have grown to love this place and its environs more than I had ever thought possible. I'm lucky, too, in that once I began to go for walks again, I could access the thousand-acre forested campus of the liberal arts college near us. Over recent years, I've experienced there the second-growth forest during all the seasons—rain dripping from the licorice ferns on the giant maples; creeks cutting ravines down to the salt-water bay; seagulls dropping shellfish on rocks to crack and eat them; crested kingfishers screeching, darting, and diving out over the water; great blue herons emitting their long, haunting squawks high up in the trees as they spread their huge wings for flight and soft landings along the shore.

Being in nature is the best therapy we can find. A sense of place is important to us. When we find a place in nature that feels comfortable and secure to us, that feels like "home," we can begin to become acquainted with the trees, the shrubbery, the animals who habitually move through it. We can take our dogs walking there, enjoying the companionship they provide. Or we can go alone or with friends. Meeting others along our path, we greet everyone happy to be out relishing the beauty of this natural world.

I find that I do my most creative thinking on my daily walks in the woods. I solve problems that seem insoluble away from the natural environment. I have insights that I probably would not have were I not in the woods. When I walk with friends, I feel our bonds tightening, our friendship deepening. This walking is one of the happiest times of my day. If you can walk even fifteen minutes, get a good pair of walking shoes and venture out. Leave your arms unencumbered so that they can swing at your sides. This provides an excellent opportunity for your body and mind to integrate. Out there, in the "real world," we can temporarily leave the complexities of our complicated lives. Nature walks can be life-sustaining for those of us with chronic illness. I invite you to come and walk with me. Let us leave the lupus behind, as we stride toward renewing our health.

13

How to Begin

Now that you have read this book, you may be wondering how to begin applying these alternative therapies to healing SLE. To help you get started, I have created the following road map to guide you through the approaches I discuss, with monthly signposts to help you on your way. It's important to note that the amount of time spent on each step may vary from person to person. Healing is an individual and ongoing process. Since SLE occurs on a cellular level, you will need to commit to improving your cellular health. In order to accomplish this, it is important to set four goals. First, take charge of your healing process. Second, agree to make the necessary lifestyle changes described in the book. Third, plan to spend a minimum of one year using these alternative approaches. Fourth, decide you will be methodical and patient as you travel the road to recovery.

To start using the road map, read chapter 12 again. In month one think about nurturing your spirit by changing your attitudes toward your illness. Be kind to yourself. If you are too ill to manage your SLE, ask a friend or family member to help you communicate with the alternative practitioners you choose. Believe that you can recover. Use some of the suggestions in this chapter for alleviating your loneliness and engaging in creative activity each day. Write your positive affirmations every morning. Try to spend some time in nature three times a week.

Next, in this first month explain to your family and friends the shift you are going to make in being proactive about healing your SLE. Ask them for their help and support. Begin to focus on helping your body recover. Decide to assist your liver health by putting fewer toxins into your body. To accomplish this, you will need to change the way you eat. Read chapter 3 again, paying attention to the suggestions for lowering liver stress. Begin eating more natural sodium in the form of vegetables. Slowly decrease the number of chemicals you eat. This includes processed foods and pharmaceuticals. If you need help making these transitions, consider visiting a naturopath or alternatively trained nutritionist to discuss these dietary changes. Do not drink alcohol. If you smoke, a TCM practitioner can help you stop. Ally yourself only with those practitioners you trust. Commit to turning to them throughout your healing for information and support. Avoid eating spices because they stress your liver. Eat more complex carbohydrates such as brown rice, whole grain pasta, and millet.

Staying with chapter 3, begin cutting the amount of fat and protein you eat to give your liver a rest. Use one or more of the gentle detoxifying methods described in the chapter, such as taking saunas. Also, consider taking one of the herbs listed in the chapter, such as milk thistle, for detoxifying your liver. Start with very low doses to make certain you can tolerate it. Later, try one of the Chinese herbs such as Xiao Yo Wan, and one dietary supplement such as vitamin C. Stay on this regimen for one month. If you don't feel better, remain on the modified diet and start another combination of no more than one herb and one supplement at a time. If you start to feel better, add another supplement, and another, as long as you continue to feel improvement.

During this first month start recording how you are feeling in a journal. Has your health improved in any way? If so, be sure you document those specific improvements. Reading your journal pages occasionally will help you stay on the journey to renewed health. If you are not improving, don't be discouraged. One month is a short time for your body to adjust to these dietary and lifestyle changes. Be willing to give it more time. Faithfully write the affirmation ten times a day, "I am helping my body to recover from lupus."

In the second month, try more dietary changes. Read chapter 4 again, and begin incorporating the suggestions found there. Continue eating more natural sodium in alkaline vegetable broths. Be sure you're drinking eight to ten glasses of water each day. This can include fresh vegetable juice. Stop drinking coffee, tea, and cola. Continue to avoid alcohol. Stop eating alfalfa sprouts. Also, remove sugar in all its forms from your diet. Instead, use the non-sugar sweeteners mentioned in the chapter.

The road map takes you farther still into the nutritional landscape this month. Read chapter 7 again, making sure you understand the importance of eating the right oils to recover from chronic illness. Reduce the saturated animal fat in your diet as much as possible and begin to eat the omega-9 monounsaturated oils such as olive, canola, and peanut. Eat cold-water, fatty fish twice a week for the essential fatty acids (EFAs) fish provides. Also, eat one of the oils that supplies the essential fatty acids LA and LNA. These EFAs may help correct immune dysfunction, and they may lower your pain level as well. Continue all these dietary improvements, and continue spending time in nature, walking or gardening, if possible. Record any changes in your symptoms in your journal.

During the third month, make certain you understand the section on GLA in chapter 7. Add a GLA supplement to your nutritional regimen if you think your symptoms might be helped by it. Then read chapter 8 again to remind yourself that our food supply is contaminated with toxic chemicals from pesticides. Begin eating as much organic food as possible. If you are unable to eat a totally organic diet, at least stop eating supermarket apples, peaches, winter squash, green beans, pears, spinach, and grapes. These fresh foods have the highest measured toxicity scores, and should be purchased only from organic sources. Cut back drastically on eating processed foods to avoid the potentially toxic additives they contain. Eat only organic meat and dairy products to avoid toxic chemical residues, which are often present in these foods.

Now that you have improved your diet, at the beginning of the fourth month, the map next points to the peaceful, rolling hills of your mind/body connection. Read chapter 11 again. Focus on letting your spirit help you to heal. Make a point of listening to music that helps you relax and feel happier. Eventually incorporate some simple body movement, taking care to adjust it to your level of illness. If you are seriously ill with SLE, walking for ten minutes may be your limit; if your illness is less severe, begin some simple tai chi, yoga, or free-form dance. Definitely learn one of the breathing exercises and perform it at least once a day. Consider one of the therapies mentioned in the chapter: hypnosis, NLP, and biofeedback. Make a decision to start one of these therapies in the fourth or fifth month, if it seems appropriate. Learn the progressive relaxation exercise in this chapter and perform it faithfully once a day. Continue to keep your journal, recording your thoughts about yourself and your illness. Are you feeling better? Praise and thank yourself for being proactive in treating your disease. Write the following affirmation ten times every day: "I am in charge of improving my health."

By the fifth month you are eating correctly for healing, exercising moderately, and thinking positively about your recovery. At this point you may have the energy and interest to begin reaching out to environmental, spiritual, or alternative health groups with which you can find a sense of community and support. Read chapter 5 again. It's time to begin trying additional nutritional supplements, including herbs that may give your body the boost it needs. Study the chapter carefully. Read about biochemic tissue salts and glandular extracts. If either of these approaches sounds reasonable to you, start using one carefully. Also add one or two of the nine supplements described in chapter 5 to your daily program. Read chapter 6 again and decide to take one of the herbal formulas that can serve as an immunomodulator, calming an overactive immune system. If you are still fatigued, consider using one of the ginsengs for no longer than two months to raise your energy level.

During this month review chapter 10 again. If you are comfortable with the TCM approach, make an appointment to visit a licensed TCM practitioner and discuss your SLE symptoms in the context of therapeutic herbs and acupuncture. Be sure you find a practitioner who uses Chinese herbs in his or her treatment protocols. Be willing to try a Chinese patent medicine for a minimum of six weeks, if you can tolerate it. Work the acupressure points described in chapter 10 for relieving lupus symptoms. Do this each day for a minimum of two months to measure adequately whether acupressure helps you. Continue to use your journal for writing and reflection. Stay with the therapies that seem to be diminishing your SLE symptoms. If you are not feeling better, change the supplements you are taking, using some of the others mentioned in chapters 3, 5, and 6. It is important to continue eating correctly, exercising, and thinking affirmatively about your recovery. Be sure you write affirmations every day.

In the sixth month the road map brings you to a steep hill. To navigate it, read chapter 9 again. By this time, you may be strong enough to consider removal of the mercury amalgams in your teeth. If you are not well enough yet, wait until twelve months have passed. Meanwhile, one of the most important steps you can take to protect your immune system is to refuse to allow your dentist to place more mercury amalgams in your mouth. If you have a large number of amalgams, particularly fillings that are less than ten years old, start taking selenium, magnesium, glutathione, zinc, B_1, and B complex at the doses recommended in chapter 9. Find a dentist who has training in amalgam removal. Have an amalgameter reading and talk with the dentist about sequential removal of your dental fillings. If you are strong enough to go through the dental procedures, have all your amalgams removed sequentially over a period of months. Bonded resins should be used as replacement materials. You may also need to have crowns replaced with porcelain or gold if your original crowns contain metal liners made with nickel, copper, or metal alloys.

Spend the next six months learning how to coordinate and regularly practice all the healing techniques you've found to be helpful in the first six months. Depending on the severity of your illness, the goals of the first six months may take you a year to complete. Move through the healing suggestions consciously and gradually, remaining sensitive to your personal needs and abilities. Continue balancing the therapies, increasing your physical and creative activities over time as your body and energy allow, and be sure to write affirmations and entries in your healing journal every day. Remember to continue integrating the mind-body therapies described in chapter 11 into your daily life. Most important, tend your spirit in all the ways discussed in chapter 12.

At the end of the first year, take stock of how you're feeling. Be proud of your efforts. Give a party for yourself and the people who have helped you. Continue these alternative approaches to healing over many years, always taking care to follow the stress reduction approaches you have learned. If you're only slightly better after one year, decide that more time devoted to using these alternative therapies will help you. Stay with it. Never give up. Always believe your health will improve. I hope the information in this book assists you in your recovery from SLE.

Epilogue

I am walking below a many-tiered canopy of ancient cedar, hemlock, and Douglas fir trees. Club moss drapes from their limbs like thick, shaggy hair. This is the heart of the Olympic rain forest, which some winters absorbs up to fifteen feet of rain. But on this lovely July day there is no dampness, and I have no need of rain gear. The trail is wide and sloping, bringing small groups of smiling day hikers toward me. We are walking through one of the last fragments of temperate rain forest on the planet. The air we are breathing is some of the purest on earth.

I know that this trail was cut in the late 1800s, long before these aged forests were granted protection by Congress under the Roosevelt Administration in 1938. Today this northwestern corner of the United States not only is managed as Olympic National Park but also carries the designation of Biosphere Reserve and World Heritage Site. These one million acres are recognized as a superb ecosystem found nowhere else in the world. Biologists acknowledge that they cannot completely comprehend the complexity of the interdependent web of life they find here.

I've been in this wilderness for a week now, hiking these mountains, ravines, and riverbanks with people from all over the United States. After months of dense, low clouds and constant rain, the weather finally has reversed for us, and sun begins to spatter these splendid trees and dapple the lakes and rivers visible from the high lookout points. We can see far up into British Columbia, up to the snow-covered Coast Ranges. The opening to the Strait of Juan de Fuca is even visible, where early Spanish and Portuguese sailing ships wrecked in fierce storms and thick fog.

It is good to be here. Yesterday my legs carried me seven miles through the Sol Duc River Valley. Tomorrow they will boost me up six miles of trail to Hurricane Ridge at 5,900 feet. I have managed every hike. Although I am tired and missing my afternoon rests, I still am able to trek up steep grades, even late in the day. I'm enjoying hiking with these robust, ebullient people, but this afternoon I feel the need to leave the group and walk on by myself.

As I pace ahead toward the waterfall, I am aware of being completely alone for the first time in a week. How different this solitude is for me now than it used to be. During the worst years of the lupus, I was terrified of being alone, even in my own home. Now I'm striding contentedly along, greeting other hikers, but feeling no need to join them. As I walk, I marvel at these 150-foot-high western red cedars and 200-foot-high Douglas firs, all hundreds of years old. Their massive height is cushioned by an understory of sword fern, evergreen huckleberry, wood sorrel, mosses, and herbs. I know spotted owls live here, but I have never seen or heard one. The music of a tiny winter wren's 102-note song surrounds me. Two octaves below that melody I hear the river drumming to the east.

This is my temple, my mosque, my cathedral, my kiva—the most spiritual place on earth for me. This is where I imagine I hear the uilleann pipes, the bamboo flute, the thumb piano, the vibrating pipe organ, the didgeridoo. Here I experience what the Buddha must have meant when he said, "I am awake." I have longed for this place for more than fourteen years, doing everything I could to regain enough physical strength to return to this wilderness, but wondering whether I would ever experience it again. And now I am here—the thunderous waterfall misting my hair and eyelashes, moistening my binoculars as I scan for water ouzels below the falls. I am dabbing tears of gratitude as I descend the mountain.

At a fork in the trail I see a signpost that reads, "Lookout Ridge, 6.5 miles. Trail Unmaintained." I learned from a park ranger that morning that this is an old Department of Interior trail cut in the early 1900s when the government was surveying the Olympic Mountains. Much of this country still has not been surveyed. I know that even well-maintained park trails can be treacherous. Just two days earlier, a woman hiking with our group lost her footing and tumbled forty feet, seriously injuring her leg. Our guide said she was lucky to be alive. "What would this unmaintained trail be like?" I wonder. "Well," I think, "this could be a test of whether I can actually hike a steep, rooted, overgrown trail by myself. Should I try it?" Alhough I am aware of many reasons not to start up the trail, I make the decision to go ahead.

As the angle steepens, I can feel my thigh and calf muscles beginning to strain. A few hundred yards and my heart is already pounding. "Good," I think. "Now I'm getting some aerobic benefit. If my knees hold out, I can keep going." I remember to look behind me often, since we've been told of fresh cougar scat found in the area. Huge, stealthy cats, they have been known to attack from behind with no warning. "What if I meet a cougar here?" I wonder. "I'm moving so far away from the main trail that no one will hear my screams. There's no one hiking up here who would find me. But this is so beautiful, I want to continue."

An hour of steady uphill hiking brings me to a massive, hand-built bridge constructed by the Civilian Conservation Corps in the 1930s. It seems strange to find something built by human hands so far up here. How did they stretch these rough-hewn, heavy beams so high over this ravine? I dangle my feet over the edge of the bridge, open my canteen, and begin thinking about how I got here.

During the years when my lupus was severe, I could not have imagined sitting alone on this bridge in this wilderness. I had panic attacks nearly every day, sometimes even when I was just lying in bed. The panic syndrome drove me into agoraphobia, the fear of leaving my house. I was afraid that if I had a panic attack "out there," I couldn't get back to safety. Even worse were the physical symptoms of the illness. After five years of debilitation, when the lupus tests were finally performed, they showed that my immune system was attacking my striated muscle tissue. The muscle weakness was so deep that I could not walk normally. At times I could not even feed myself. My immune system also was attacking my heart muscle, and I was told by medical personnel that my heart had been severely affected. Although I couldn't feel my heart's weakness, I often had heart palpitations that drove me into emergency rooms more than once.

During those years, I was so thin that much of my skeletal structure was visible. At five feet, eight inches, I weighed only 112 pounds. Vertigo forced me to hold on to walls to walk, and I could not look at the beautiful Douglas fir trees outside our home because they seemed to be closing in on me. I was so claustrophobic that I couldn't stay in closed rooms or dense forests. My fatigue never abated. I could visit with friends and family only an hour at a time before I became exhausted and needed rest. I was in such constant joint and muscle pain that I needed help dressing myself. I could not sew, could not plant or weed my gardens, could not even stand in the kitchen and chop vegetables. My vision was so cloudy that I could not see well enough to read. The brain fog I endured kept me from understanding what people were saying to me. I could not hear a paragraph from a book and fully understand it. My hearing was muffled. A constant low-grade fever left me feeling as though I were burning up.

Resting now on this old bridge, I am completely alone, and I am cherishing these moments. Being here is proof, I think, that recent blood tests are correct—that the level of autoimmune attack in my body is greatly reduced from five or ten years ago. With diminishing levels of attack on my body tissue, I am able to function again. My muscles are strong now from the one to three miles I have walked nearly every day for the past five years. Even though my heart has been pounding from this rapid elevation gain, medical tests show that my heart muscle is quite strong. Now that I have gained weight, I feel that my body is strong enough to carry me through physical challenges. The vertigo has vanished. I can look up at the tree canopy and not feel it moving toward me. My cloudy vision and muffled hearing have cleared, allowing me to see the details of the vegetation around me and hear the timbre of the river's rushing waters.

My claustrophobia, I realize, has disappeared; I can walk in this dense forest breathing deeply and thinking calmly. I am tired from the exertion of climbing up this ravine. Although I know that my energy level is still not what it was before the illness, I also know that I can move quickly through this forest if I need to. I am very hot now, but the heat is from this sweltering July day, not the low-grade fever that burdened me for years. Today my joint and muscle pain has lessened. I am still in pain, but I can manage it. Best of all, I'm thinking clearly and positively enough to have made the decision to take this trail.

Beyond this comfortable spot above the river, I begin to inventory the activities I can participate in again. I have been able to ride in the car for long trips—one thousand miles to northern British Columbia, two thousand miles to Glacier National Park. I am driving again, though I still fatigue easily and cannot manage the speed and frenzy of the freeways. I am Nordic-skiing now, though I can do so for only one hour at a time. I can cook and sew and sing and play the piano. And I can engage in one of my most cherished activities—gardening. Soon I will rise into the stratosphere on my first jumbo jet flight in fourteen years. Finally, I can comprehend what people say to me. I can read challenging books again and understand them.

By adhering to a schedule of regular rest, I am able to take an active part in community life once more. I mentor environmental study groups in our city and work as a Stream Team volunteer, helping restore natural habitat for the wild Pacific salmon returning to spawn. I participate in a book discussion group. I am able to give an occasional small party. I can attend concerts and even do a bit of pencil drawing.

The years of searching for natural healing therapies have rewarded me. My camels have returned to their desert home because I no longer need to go out on safari. I still see the images of the Karamojong tribesmen, but their colors are softer, their words far less urgent. Together we have banished the lupus wolf from my door. He has gone back to the mountains, and I have remained here, beginning to experience once again the richness of a life I cherish. People around me express their delight that I am recovering. One of my best friends says that there is nothing sweeter than the sound of my rekindled laughter. My husband says that there is nothing sweeter than my regained ability to accompany him into the wilderness.

And my mother says that there is nothing sweeter than my writing this book.

Resting now from the day's strenuous hike, I am sitting cross-legged on the shore of Lake Crescent. The beauty of this glacier-fed lake surrounded by forested mountains touches my soul. I feel completely melded with this place. Taking my notebook from my pack, I begin writing . . .

> *In this moment,*
> *The silky, teal waves chatter like shell rattles*
> *beneath the feather-textured mountains.*
> *I am trout-woman, my body shimmering*
> *green and magenta, my fins like bows on a silky dress.*
> *My ears are gills picking up staccato sounds*
> *as I move below the white noise of the surface.*
> *I am wild—wild as the Orcas of Puget Sound,*
> *wild as the gorillas of the Mountains of the Moon,*
> *wild as the polar bears of the northern ice.*
> *And I am safe—surrounded by softness—as I glide*
> *the havens of weather-smooth, water-dense snags.*

I read what I've written. My words reveal a mind well enough at last to move beyond illness, to think creatively again. And I rejoice.

Suggested Reading

Conventional Medicine

Dibner, Robin, and Carol Colman. *Lupus Handbook for Women*. New York: Fireside, 1994.

Horowitz, Mark, and Marietta Abrams Brill. *Living with Lupus: A Comprehensive Guide to Understanding and Controlling Lupus While Getting On with Your Life*. New York: Penguin Books, 1994.

Wallace, Daniel. *The Lupus Book: A Guide for Patients and Their Families*. New York: Oxford University Press, 1995.

Fats and Oils

Erasmus, Udo. *Fats and Oils: A Complete Guide to Fats and Oils in Health and Nutrition*. Burnaby, B.C., Canada: Alice Books, 1986.

Murray, Michael T. *Understanding Fats and Oils*. Encinitas, Calif.: Progressive Health Publishing, 1996.

Food Toxins

Blaylock, Russell L. *Excitotoxins*. Santa Fe: Health Press, 1994.

Colburn, Theo, Dianne Dumanoski, and John Peterson Myers. *Our Stolen Future*. New York: Dutton, 1996.

Robbins, John. *Diet for a New America*. Tiburon, Calif.: H. J. Kramer, 1987.

General Healing

Golan, Ralph. *Optimal Wellness*. New York: Ballantine Books, 1995.

Pizzorno, Joseph, and Michael Murray. *Encyclopedia of Natural Health*. Rocklin, Calif.: Prima Publishing, 1990.

Weil, Andrew. *Spontaneous Healing*. New York: Ballantine Books, 1995.

Herbs

Hobbs, Christopher. *Foundations of Health: The Liver and Digestive Herbal.* Capitola, Calif.: Botanical Press, 1992.

Murray, Michael. *The Healing Power of Herbs.* Rocklin, Calif.: Prima Publishing, 1995.

Mind–Body Awareness

Dossey, Larry. *Prayer Is Good Medicine.* New York: Harper, 1996.

Emerick, John J., Jr. *Be the Person You Want to Be: Harness the Power of Neurolinguistic Programming to Reach Your Potential.* Rocklin, Calif.: Prima Publishing, 1997.

Hendricks, Gay. *Conscious Breathing: Breathwork for Health, Stress Release, and Personal Mastery.* New York: Bantam Books, 1995.

Kabat-Zinn, Jon. *Full Catastrophe Living: Using the Wisdom of Your Body and Mind to Face Stress, Pain, and Illness.* New York: Delta, 1990.

Nutrition

Calbom, Cherie, and Maureen Keane. *Juicing for Life.* New York: Avery Publishing Group, 1992.

Holford, Patrick. *Optimum Nutrition Bible.* Freedom, Calif.: Crossing Press, 1999.

Kushi, Michio. *Holistic Health through Macrobiotics: Complete Guide to Mind–Body Healing.* New York: Farrar, Straus, and Giroux, 1993.

Leighton, Steward, H., et al. *Sugar Busters: Cut Sugar to Trim Fat.* New York: Ballantine Books, 1998.

Pitchford, Paul. *Healing with Whole Foods: Oriental Traditions and Modern Nutrition.* Berkeley, Calif.: North Atlantic Books, 1993.

Traditional Chinese Medicine

Elias, Jason, and Katherine Ketcham. *The Five Elements of Self-Healing.* New York: Harmony Books, 1998.

Liu, Henry B. *Chinese Health Secrets: A Natural Lifestyle Approach.* St. Paul: Llewellyn, 2000.

Reed Gach, Michael. *Acupressure's Potent Points: A Guide to Self-Care for Common Ailments.* New York: Bantam Books, 1990.

Resources

The author would appreciate hearing from you about any alternative healing approaches that have reduced your lupus symptoms. You may contact her through her Web page at www.abouthealinglupus.com

GENERAL RESOURCES

The following Web sites are useful not only for those with SLE, but for anyone, healthy or ill, who wishes to learn more about alternative medicine.

Alternative Health News Online: www.altmedicine.com

NaturalHealthWeb.com: www.naturalhealthweb.com
> These Web sites provide both general and specific information on many of the alternative health practices discussed in this book, as well as links to other helpful sites.

Alternative Medicine Review: www.thorne.com/altmedrev/index.html
> This Web site contains updated, professional articles on the latest alternative medicine research.

National Center for Complementary and Alternative Medicine: http://nccam.nih.gov/

This Web site serves as an excellent clearinghouse and gateway to further information about alternative medicine for both consumers and practitioners.

CHAPTER RESOURCES

Chapter 8 • Environmental Toxins in Food

Community Supported Agriculture (CSA) programs are increasing in number every year in the United States. The following organization can provide free listings of CSA farms in your area. Their directory can also be viewed on their Web site.

CSA/CSREES
1400 Independence Avenue S.W.
Stop 2207
Washington, D.C. 20250-2207
www.SARE.org/san/CSA/index.htm

Chapter 9 • The Dangers of Toxic Dentistry

The following organizations can provide information about mercury amalgam removal.

Clifford Consulting and Research, Inc.
P.O. Box 17597
Colorado Springs, CO 80935-7597
(719) 550-0008
www.ccrlab.com
> This laboratory can refer you to a dentist in your area who has been trained in amalgam removal. It also provides biocompatibility tests for replacement materials.

Peak Energy Performance (PEP)

(800) 331-2303

> This laboratory provides biocompatibility tests for amalgam
> replacement.

Matrix

Gary Jacobson, D.D.S.

(877) 877-7900

> Dr. Jacobson will refer you to a dentist in your area who has
> been trained by Dr. Huggins to remove dental amalgams.

Dental Amalgam Mercury Syndrome (DAMS)

P.O. Box 64397

Virginia Beach, VA 23467-4397

(800) 311-6265

> This is a support group of patients who feel a strong dedica-
> tion to informing fellow citizens of the health hazards associ-
> ated with mercury amalgam fillings. A basic information
> packet is available from DAMS .

International Academy of Oral Medicine and Toxicology

P.O. Box 458

Ortonville, MI 48462

> This organization is able to provide the name of a dentist in
> your area who is familiar with the mercury amalgam toxicity
> issue and the correct protocols for replacement.

Chapter 10 • Traditional Chinese Medicine

*The Acuhealth home acupuncture kit can relieve a number of symptoms,
including dizziness, fatigue, and joint and muscle pain. The following company can provide information for ordering the kit.*

Acu-Medical Supplies, Ltd.
44 Royal York Road
Toronto, Canada M8V 2T4
(800) 567-7246

Chapter 12 • Caring for Your Spirit

Anyone with a debilitating illness or other physical challenge can benefit from the spirit-tending services offered by organizations such as the two that follow. There are many more such organizations—research and reach out to those located in your community.

National Library Service for the Blind and Physically Handicapped
Library of Congress
Washington, D.C. 20542
(202) 707-5100

The Delta Society
289 Parameter East
Renton, WA 98055-1329
(800) 869-6898
www.deltasociety.org
> This organization can provide information on locating a
> trained companion dog. A service dog directory can be down-
> loaded from their Web site.

Notes

Chapter 2: What Is Lupus?

1. National Institutes of Health press release, February 15, 1997.
2. Sheldon Blau, *Living with Lupus: All the Knowledge You Need to Help Yourself* (Reading, Mass.: Addison-Wesley, 1993), 50.
3. Ibid., 183.

Chapter 3: Your Liver

1. Adelle Davis, Let's Get Well (New York: Harcourt Brace Jovanovich, 1965), 170.
2. Henry G. Bieler, M.D., Food Is Your Best Medicine (New York: Ballantine, 1992), 42.
3. Christopher Hobbs, *Foundations of Health: The Liver and Digestive Herbal* (Capitola, Calif.: Botanical Press, 1992), 25.
4. Bieler, Food Is Your Best Medicine, 65.
5. U.S. Statistical Abstracts, 1984.
6. Davis, *Let's Get Well*, 173.
7. Hobbs, *Foundations of Health: The Liver and Digestive Herbal*, 29.
8. Bill Schoenbart and Ellen Shefi, *Chinese Healing Secrets* (Lincolnwood, Ill.: Publications International, Ltd., 1997), 31.
9. Michael Murray, N.D., and Joseph Pizzorno, N.D., *The Encyclopedia of Natural Health* (Rocklin, Calif.: Prima Publishing, 1990), 34–35.
10. Robert Gray, The Colon Health Handbook (Oakland, Calif.: Rockridge Publishing, 1983), 21.

11. Hobbs, Foundations of Health: The Liver and Digestive Herbal, 21–22.

12. Associated Press Release, February 22, 1998.

13. Donald Lepore, N.D., *The Ultimate Healing System* (Provo, Utah: Woodland Books, 1988), 159.

14. James Braly, M.D., *Dr. Braly's Optimum Health Program* (New York: Time Books, 1985), 112.

15. Ibid., 96.

16. Ibid., 96.

17. Steve Austin, N.D., and Cathy Hitchcock, *Breast Cancer: What You Should Know (But May Not Be Told) About Prevention, Diagnosis, and Treatment* (Rocklin, Calif.: Prima Publishing, 1994), 96.

18. Braly, *Dr. Braly's Optimum Health Program*, 116.

19. Ibid., 117.

20. Davis, *Let's Get Well*, 173.

21. Braly, *Dr. Braly's Optimum Health Program*, 188.

22. Lepore, *The Ultimate Healing System*, 173.

23. Andrew Weil, M.D., *Spontaneous Healing* (New York: Ballantine Books, 1996), 80–81.

Chapter 4: Your Diet

1. Paavo Airola, N.D., Ph.D., *How to Get Well* (Phoenix, Ariz.: Health Plus Publishers, 1975), 254.

2. Henry G. Bieler, M.D., *Food Is Your Best Medicine* (New York: Ballantine Books, 1992), 205.

3. Ibid., 206.

4. Cherie Calbom and Maureen Keane, *Juicing for Life* (New York: Avery Publishing Group, 1992), 19.

5. Ibid., 16.

6. Steven Masley, M.D., *The 28-Day Antioxidant Diet Program* (Olympia, Wash.: 1997), 77.

7. Christopher Hobbs, *Foundations of Health: The Liver and Digestive Herbal* (Capitola, Calif.: Botanical Press, 1992), 42.

8. Linda Rector-Page, N.D., *Healthy Healing: An Alternative Healing Reference* (Sonora, Calif.: Healthy Healing Publications, 1994), 86.

9. Andrew Weil, M.D., *Spontaneous Healing* (New York: Ballantine Books, 1996), 28.

10. Daniel Wallace, M.D., *The Lupus Book* (New York: Oxford University Press, 1995), 44.

11. Ibid., 177.

12. Sarah Ziegler, R.N., *Day to Day Living with Lupus* (Los Angeles, Calif.: the author, 1996), 44.

13. Bill Schoenbart and Ellen Shefi, *Chinese Healing Secrets* (Lincolnwood, Ill.: Publications International, Ltd., 1997), 41.

14. Mark Horowitz, M.D., and Marietta Abrams Brill, *Living with Lupus: A Comprehensive Guide to Understanding and Controlling Lupus While Getting on with Your Life* (New York: Penguin Books, 1994), 152.

15. James F. Balch, M.D., and Phyllis Balch, *Prescription for Nutritional Healing* (Garden City, N.Y.: Avery Publishing Group, 1997), 105–6.

16. Tori Hudson, N.D., *Women's Encyclopedia of Natural Medicine* (Los Angeles: Keats Publishing, 1999), 117–18.

17. Masley, *The 28-Day Antioxidant Diet Program,* 65.

18. Robert S. Ivker, D.O., *Sinus Survival* (New York: Putman Books, 1995), 139.

Chapter 5: Helpful Nutritional Supplements

1. "Diet and Cancer," Interview with John D. Potter, M.D., *Nutrition Action Healthletter* (Washington, D.C.: Center for Science in the Public Interest, December, 1998), 6.

2. Andrew Stanway, *Biochemic Tissue Salts* (Wellingborough, Northamptonshire, U.K.: Thorsons Publishing Group, 1987), 29.

3. F. August Luyties, *The Biochemic Handbook* (St. Louis, Mo.: Formur International, 1976).

4. James Balch, M.D., and Phyllis A. Balch, *Prescription for Nutritional Healing* Garden City, N.Y.: Avery Publishing Group, 1997), 550.

5. Ibid., 552.

6. James Braly, M.D., *Dr. Braly's Optimum Health Program* (New York: Time Books, 1985), 156.

7. Ralph Golan, M.D., *Optimal Wellness* (New York: Ballantine Books, 1995), 134.

8. Michael Murray, N.D., and Joseph Pizzorno, N.D., *The Encyclopedia of Natural Health* (Rocklin, Calif.: Prima Publishing, 1990), 64.

9. "Effect of Vitamin A Treatment on the Immune Reactivity of Patients with Systemic Lupus Erythematosus," *Journal of Clinical Laboratory Immunology* 26 (1988), 33–35.

10. Cherie Calbom and Maureen Keane, *Juicing For Life* (New York: Avery Publishing Group, 1992), 19.

11. Lendon Smith, *Feed Yourself Right* (New York: Dell Trade Paperback, 1983), 304.

12. G. Lenaz, *Coenzyme Q-10: Biochemistry, Bioenergetics and Clinical Applications of Ubiquinone* (New York: John Wiley and Sons, 1985).

13. Michael Murray and Joseph Pizzorno, *The Encyclopedia of Natural Medicine*, 496.

14. Patricia Slagle, M.D., *How to Get Up from Down* (New York: Random House, 1987), 43–45.

15. Dean Ward, M.D., *Smart Drugs and Nutrients* (Menlo Park, Calif.: Health Freedom Publications, 1990), 95.

16. Ibid., 81.

17. Alan Gaby, M.D., "DHEA: The Hormone That Does It All," *Holistic Medicine* Spring 1993, 20.

18. A. G. Schwartz et al., "Dehydroepiandrosterone and Structural Analogs," *Advances in Cancer Research* 51 (1988): 391–424.

19. "DHEA Gets Respect," *Harvard Healthletter* 19 (July, 1994).

20. "Dehydroepiandrosterone," *Journal of Clinical Endocrinology and Metabolism* 29, no. 2 (February 1969): 273–78.

21. R. F. van Vollenhoven et al., "An Open Study of Dehydroepiandrosterone in Systemic Lupus Erythematosus," *Arthritis and Rheumatism* 37, no. 9 (September 1994): 1305–10.

22. Alan Gaby, M.D., *Preventing and Reversing Osteoporosis* (Rocklin, Calif.: Prima Publishing, 1994), 165.

23. Ibid., 166.

Chapter 6: Healing Herbs

1. N. Farnsworth et al., "Medicinal Plants in Therapy," *Bulletin of the World Health Organization* 63 (1985), 965–81.

2. Herbal Gram 17 (1988): 16–17.

3. John Greenwald, "Herbal Healing," Time, November 23, 1998, 59.

4. Jack Challen, "The Problem with Herbs," *Natural Health,* January/February 1999, 58.

5. David Hoffman, *An Elders' Herbal* (Rochester, Vt.: Healing Arts Press, 1993), 172.

6. Michael Murray, *The Healing Power of Herbs* (Rocklin, Calif.: Prima Publishing, 1995), 5.

7. Hoffman, *An Elders' Herbal,* 174.

8. D. Vensky and A. Gamble, *Chinese Herbal Medicine: Materia Medica* (Seattle, Wash.: Eastland Press, 1986), 83.

9. Christopher Hobbs, *Foundations of Health: The Liver and Digestive Herbal* (Capitola, Calif.: Botanical Press, 1992), 284.

10. Hoffman, *An Elders' Herbal,* 204.

11. Michael Tierra, N.D., *Planetary Herbology* (Twin Lakes, Wis.: Lotus Press, 1988), 309.

12. Murray, *The Healing Power of Herbs,* 175–76.

13. Hoffman, *An Elders' Herbal,* 247.

14. Ibid., 185.

15. "Hypericum Research Continues," International Phytomedicine Conference Report, part 1, *Medi Herb Monitor,* November 19, 1996, 12.

16. Ibid., 14.

17. Christopher Hobbs, *The Ginsengs* (Santa Cruz, Calif.: Botanica Press, 1996), 15.

18. Ibid., 60–61.

19. D. E. Moerman, *Medicinal Plants of Native Americans* (Ann Arbor, Mich.: Regents of the University of Michigan, 1986), 87.

20. Hobbs, *The Ginsengs,* 69.

21. *Naturopathic Treatment Notebook* (Seattle, Wash.: Bastyr College of Natural Health Sciences, 1984).

22. Harper-Shore, IBIS Database, Seattle, Wash.: University of Washington Health Sciences Library, April 1999.

23. *National College of Naturopathic Medicine Clinical Notes* (Portland, Ore., 1984–1991).

24. Anderson and Geller, IBIS Database, Seattle, Wash.: University of Washington Health Sciences Library, April 1999.

Chapter 7: Beneficial Fats And Oils

1. Udo Erasmus, *Fats and Oils: A Complete Guide to Fats and Oils in Health and Nutrition* (Burnaby, Canada: Alive Books 1986), 168.

2. Andrew Weil, M.D., *Spontaneous Healing* (New York: Ballantine Books, 1996), 140.

3. E. J. Masoro, "Assessment of Nutritional Components in Prolongation of Life and Health by Diet," *Proceedings of the Society for Experimental Biology and Medicine* 193 (1990): 31–34.

4. Bob Arnot, M.D., *The Breast Cancer Prevention Diet* (New York: Little, Brown and Company, 1998), 69.

5. Weil, *Spontaneous Healing,* 141.

6. Arnot, *The Breast Cancer Prevention Diet,* 69.

7. Michael T. Murray, N.D., *Understanding Fats and Oils* (Encinitas, Calif.: Progressive Health Publishing, 1996), 11.

8. Erasmus, *Fats and Oils: A Complete Guide to Fats and Oils in Health and Nutrition,* 245.

9. James Braly, M.D., *Dr. Braly's Optimum Health Program* (New York: Time Books, 1985), 193.

10. Ralph Golan, M.D., *Optimal Wellness* (New York: Ballantine Books, 1995), 311.

11. Johanna Budwig, M.D., *Flax Oil as a True Aid Against Arthritis, Heart Infarction, Cancer and Other Diseases* (Vancouver, Canada: Apple Publishing Company, 1992), 31.

12. Paul Pitchford, *Healing with Whole Foods: Oriental Traditions and Modern Nutrition* (Berkeley, Calif.: North Atlantic Books, 1993), 125.

13. Richard Passwater, *Evening Primrose Oil* (New Canaan, Conn: Keats Publishing, 1981), 15.

14. Ibid., 2.

15. Erasmus, *Fats and Oils: A Complete Guide to Fats and Oils in Health and Nutrition*, 352–53.

16. Passwater, *Evening Primrose Oil*, 3.

17. Murray, *Understanding Fats and Oils*, 24.

18. Erasmus, *Fats and Oils: A Complete Guide to Fats and Oils in Health and Nutrition*, 253.

19. Passwater, *Evening Primrose Oil*, 29.

20. Murray, *Understanding Fats and Oils*, 24.

21. Braly, *Dr. Braly's Optimum Health Program*, 156.

22. Murray, *Understanding Fats and Oils*, 4–5.

23. Arnot, *The Breast Cancer Prevention Diet*, 76.

Chapter 8: Environmental Toxins in Food

1. Arun P. Kulkarni and Mitra Ashole, "Pesticide Contamination of Food in the United States," *Food Contamination from Environmental Sources* (New York: John Wiley and Sons, Inc., 1990), 264.

2. T. Vial, B. Nicolaus, and J. Descotes, "Clinical Immunotoxicity of Pesticides," *Journal of Toxicology and Environmental Health* 48, no. 3 (1996), 215–29.

3. Theo Colborn, Dianne Dumanoski, and John Peterson Myers, *Our Stolen Future* (New York: Dutton, 1996), 167.

4. Kulkarni and Ashole, "Pesticide Contamination of Food in the United States," 267.

5. Andrew Weil, M.D., *Spontaneous Healing* (New York: Ballantine Books, 1996), 133.

6. Bruce Mohl, "Illness Rates Prompt Study in South Boston," *Boston Globe* December 18, 1998.

7. Weil, *Spontaneous Healing*, 133.

8. Congress of the United States, "Environmental Contaminants in Food" (Washington, D.C.: Office of Technology Assessment, December, 1979), 59–61.

9. Commission on Life Science, National Research Council, *Pesticides in the Diets of Infants and Children* (Washington, D.C: National Academy Press, 1993), 240.

10. Ruth Lowengart et al., "Childhood Leukemia and Parents' Occupational and

Home Exposures," *Journal of National Cancer Institute* 79 (1987): 39–46.

11. Commission on Life Science, *Pesticides in the Diets of Infants and Children,* 67.

12. Ibid., 69.

13. Ibid., 109.

14. P. Thomas, H. Ratajczak, D. Demetral, K. Hagen, and R. Baron, "Aldicarb Immunotoxicity: Functional Analysis of Cell-mediated Immunity and Quantition of Lymphocyte Subpopulations," *Fundamental and Applied Toxicology* 15 (1990) 221–230.

15. Lawrie Mott and Karen Snyder, *Pesticide Alert* (Washington, D.C.: Natural Resources Defense Council, 1987), 20.

16. Ibid., 12–15.

17. "How Safe Is Our Produce?" *Consumer Reports* March 1999, 28–31.

18. Annette Pernelle Hoyer et al., "Organochlorine Exposure and Risk of Breast Cancer," *Lancet* 352 (December 5, 1998) 1816–20.

19. *Nutrition Action Healthletter* (Washington, D.C.: Center for Science in the Public Interest, March 1998), 8.

20. Michael H. Thomas, "Drug Residues in Animal Tissues," *Journal of the Association of Analytical Chemistry* 72 (July/August, 1989), 533.

21. Ibid.

22. "Organic Food Program," Washington State Department of Agriculture Bulletin, 1998.

23. "How Safe Is Our Produce?" 28–31.

24. Russell L. Blaylock, M.D., *Excitotoxins* (Santa Fe, N.M.: Health Press, 1994), 125, 215.

25. Ibid., 16.

26. Ibid., 16.

27. M. Kubera et al., "Effect of Monosodium Glutamate on Cell-mediated Immunity," *Polish Journal of Pharmacology and Pharmacy* 43(1991), 39–44.

28. "Chemical Cuisine," *Nutrition Action Healthletter,* (Washington, D.C.: Center for Science in the Public Interest, (March 1999), 4–8.

29. Colborn, Dumanoski, and Myers, *Our Stolen Future,* 214.

30. Congress of the United States, Subcommittee on Oversight and Investigations, *Cancer-Causing Chemicals in Food,* December 1978 (Washington, D.C.: House Interstate and Foreign Commerce Committee), 25.

31. Orville Schell, *Modern Meat* (New York: Random House, 1984), 327.

32. Ibid., 11.

33. Ibid., 190.

34. Ibid., 252.

35. Colborn, Dumanoski, and Myers, *Our Stolen Future*, 63.

36. M. J. Rood, et al., " Female Sex Hormones at the Onset of Systemic Lupus Erythematosus Affect Survival," *British Journal of Rheumatology* 37, no. 9 (1998), 1008–10.

37. Schell, *Modern Meat*, 291.

38. John Robbins, *Diet for a New America* (Tiburon, Calif.: H. J. Kramer, 1987), 328.

39. "Dioxin Contamination of Milk," testimony of Mark Floegel, Hearing Before the Subcommittee on Health and the Environment of the Committee on Energy and Commerce, U.S. House of Representatives, September 8, 1989, 16–19.

40. "National Wildlife Federation Sues EPA over Paper-mill Pollution Rules," *National Wildlife* August 1998, 64.

41. Lewis Regenstein, *America the Poisoned* (Washington, D.C.: Acropolis Books, Ltd., 1982), 336.

42. Ibid., 334.

43. Toxaphene Working Group, "Toxaphene: Position Document 1" (Washington, D.C.: Environmental Protection Agency, April 19, 1977), 19.

44. J. Mason and P. Singer, *Animal Factories* (New York: Crown Publishers, 1980), 56–58.

45. Joel Salatin *Pastured Poultry Profits* (Swoope, Va.: Polyface, 1993).

Chapter 9: The Dangers of Toxic Dentistry

1. *Townsend Letter for Doctors and Patients*, August 9, 1992, cited in *Spectrum*, December 12, 1992: 19–20,27.

2. Hal A. Huggins, D.D S , *It's All in Your Head* (Nashville, Tenn.: Winston Derek, 1985), 142.

3. A. Stock, *Chronisch Queksilber und Amalgam Vergiftung*, Zahnarztl: Rundschau 48 (1939), 403.

4. "Amalgam Declared Hazardous," *Dentistry Today*, February 1989, 1.

5. "Mercury Free and Healthy: The Dental Amalgam Issue," www.amalgam.org, 1996: 16.

6. Keith W. Sehnert, M.D., Gary Jacobson, D.D.S., and Kip Sullivan, "Is Mercury Toxicity an Autoimmune Disorder?" www.thorne.com/townsend/oct/mercury.html, June 26, 1999, 3.

7. Thomas B. Eyl, M.D., "Methyl Mercury Poisoning in Fish and Human Beings," *Modern Medicine* November 16, 1970, 135–36.

8. Huggins, *It's All in Your Head*, 28.

9. Patrick Stortebecker, M.D., Mercury Poisoning from Dental Amalgam—A Hazard to Human Brain (Orlando, Fl.: Bio-Probe, 1985), 164.

10. R. L. Siblerud, "Relationship Between Mercury from Dental Amalgam and Health," *Toxic Substances Journal* 10 (1990), 425–44.

11. C. K. Blesius, E. Del Vall, and D. Clason, "Dental Amalgam and Mercury," *Townsend Letter for Doctors and Patients* October 31, 1996, 86–91.

12. Sam Ziff and Michael Ziff, D.D.S., *Infertility and Birth Defects: Is Mercury from Silver Dental Fillings an Unsuspected Cause?* (Orlando, Fla.: Bio-Probe, 1987), 90–93.

13. M. Nylander, L. Friberg, B. Lind, "Mercury Concentrations in the Human Brain and Kidneys in Relation to Exposure from Dental Amalgam Fillings," *Swedish Dental Journal* 1987;11:179–87.

14. Hal A. Huggins, "Results of the Coors Blood Chemistry Study on the Effects of Dental Mercury Amalgam Fillings and Recent Investigations into the Toxicity of Root Canals and Cavitations," *Townsend Letter for Doctors and Patients,* July 31, 1991, 84–85.

15. David W. Eggleston, "Effect of Dental Amalgam and Nickel Alloys on T-Lymphocytes, *Journal of Prosthetic Dentistry* 51 (1984), 619.

16. G. A. Caron, S. Poutala, and T. T. Provost, "Lymphocyte Transformation Induced by Inorganic and Organic Mercury," *International Archives of Allergy* 37 (1970), 77–78.

17. Jan Jurjen Weening, *Mercury-Induced Immune Complex Glomerulopathy: An Experimental Study,* (The Netherlands: Van Dendergen, 1980), 36–66.

18. Druet et al., "Immunologically Mediated Glomerulonephritis Induced by Heavy Metals," *Archives of Toxicology* 50 (1982), 191–92.

19. Eggleston, "Effect of Dental Amalgam and Nickle Alloys on T-Lymphocytes," 616.

20. Blesius, Del Vall, and Clason, "Dental Amalgam And Mercury," 86–91.

21. H. Hu, G. Moller, M. Abidi-Valugerdi, "Mechanism of Mercury-induced Autoimmunity: Both T Helper and T Helper 2-Type Responses Are Involved," *Immunology* 96, vol. 3 (1999), 348–57.

22. M. J. Vimy, Y. Takahashi, F. L. Lorscheider, "Maternal–Fetal Distribution of Mercury (203 Hg) Released from Dental Amalgam Fillings," *American Journal of Physiology* 258 (1990), 939–45.

23. "Mother's Dental Amalgams Associated with High Mercury Levels," *Quarterly Review of Natural Medicine* September 30, 1995, 257–58, based on original research by F. Drasch et al., "Mercury Burden of Human Fetal and Infant Tissues," *European Journal of Pediatrics* 15 (1994), 608–11.

24. Sehnert et al., "Is Mercury Toxicity an Immune Disorder?" 5.

25. L. Barregard, G. Isacsson, L. Bodin, "People with High Mercury Uptake from Their Own Dental Amalgam Fillings," *Occupational Environmental Medicine* 52 (1995), 124–28.

26. T. W. Ortendahl, P. Hogstedt, R. P. Holland, "Mercury Vapor Release from Dental Amalgam In Vitro Caused by Magnetic Fields Generated by CRTs," *Swedish Dentistry Journal* 22 (1991), 31.

27. Huggins, *It's All in Your Head*, 37.

28. Ibid., 41.

29. B. Lindqvist and H. Mornstad, "Effects of Removing Amalgam Fillings from Patients with Diseases Affecting the Immune System," *Medical Science Research* 24, vol. 5 (1996), 355–56.

30. American Dental Association Resolution 42H-1986. Transaction 1986: 536.

31. Stortebecker, *Mercury Poisoning from Dental Amalgam—A Hazard to Human Brain*, 30.

32. Ziff and Ziff, *Infertility and Birth Defects: Is Mercury from Silver Dental Fillings an Unsuspected Cause?* 112.

33. Ibid., 317.

34. Ibid., 317.

35. Morton Walker, D.P.M., *The Chelation Answer* (New York: M. Evans and Company, 1982), 31.

Chapter 10: Traditional Chinese Medicine

1. Ted J. Kaptchuk, O.M.D., *The Web That Has No Weaver: Understanding*

Chinese Medicine (New York: Congdon and Weed, Inc., 1983), 161–62.

2. Peter Firebrace and Sandra Hill, Acupuncture: How It Works, How It Cures (New Canaan, Conn.: Keats Publishing, 1994), 9–11.

3. Gary F. Fleischman, Acupuncture: Everything You Ever Wanted to Know (New York: Barrytown, Ltd., 1998), 146.

4. The Burton Goldberg Group, *Alternative Medicine: The Definitive Guide* (Fife, Wash.: Future Medicine Publishing, 1997), 37–46.

5. Personal interview with Anne Christiansen, N.D., L.Ac., April 1997.

6. M. M. Van Benschoten, "Acupoint Diagnostics and Autoimmune Disease," *American Journal of Acupuncture* 23, no. 2 (1995), 169.

7. Ibid.

8. Bob Flaws and Honora Lee Wolfe, *Prince Wen Hui's Cook: Chinese Dietary Therapy* (Brookline, Mass.: Paradigm Publications, 1983), 67.

9. Fleischman, *Acupuncture: Everything You Ever Wanted to Know,* 146.

10. Jason Elias, and Katherine Ketcham, *The Five Elements of Self-Healing* (New York: Harmony Books, 1998), 301.

11. Ibid., 302.

12. "Treatment of Systemic Lupus Erythematosus with Combined Traditional Chinese and Western Medicine," *Shanghai Journal of Traditional Chinese Medicine* 84 (1979), 22–26.

13. Feng Shu-fang, Fang Li et al., "Treatment of Systemic Lupus Erythematosus by Acupuncture," *Chinese Medical Journal* 98, vol. 3 (1985), 171–76.

14. Cheryl Schwartz, D.V.M., "Treatment of Systemic Lupus Erythematosus with Acupuncture, Chinese Herbs and Homeopathy in a Dog: A Case Report," *American Journal of Acupuncture* (1990), 247–49.

15. Daniel J. Wallace, M.D., *The Lupus Book* (New York: Oxford University Press, 1995), 191.

16. Personal interview with Anne Christiansen, N.D., L.Ac., April 1997.

17. Margaret Naeser, Ph.D., *Outline Guide to Chinese Herbal Patent Medicines* (Boston, Mass.: Boston Chinese Medicine, 1990), 20–21.

18. Ibid., 22–23.

19. Jong-Rern Chen et al., "The Effects of Chinese Herbs on Improving Survival and Inhibiting Anti-ds DNA Antibody Production in Lupus Mice." *American Journal of Chinese Medicine* 21, vol. 3–4, 257–62.

20. "Treatment of Systemic Lupus Erythematosus with Combined Traditional Chinese and Western Medicine," 22–26.

21. Naeser, *Outline Guide to Chinese Herbal Patent Medicines,* 227.

22. Elias and Ketcham, *The Five Elements of Self-Healing,* 307.

23. Henry C. Lu, *Legendary Chinese Healing Herbs* (New York: Sterling Publishing Company, 1991), 58.

24. Ibid., 146.

25. Sheldon Blau, M.D., *Living with Lupus: All the Knowledge You Need to Help Yourself* (Reading, Mass.: Addison-Wesley, 1993), 217.

26. Elias and Ketcham, *The Five Elements of Self-Healing,* 309–10.

27. Flaws and Wolfe, *Prince Wen Hui's Cook: Chinese Dietary Therapy,* 109.

28. Personal interview with Anne Christiansen, N.D., L.Ac., April 1997.

29. Miriam Lee, *Insights of a Senior Acupuncturist* (Boulder, Colo.: Blue Poppy Press, 1992), xi–xii.

Chapter 11: Mind–Body Therapies

1. Don Campbell, "The Riddle of the Mozart Effect," Natural Health, January–February, 1998, 114.

2. Andrew Weil, M.D., *Spontaneous Healing* (New York: Ballantine Books, 1996), 204.

3. Ibid., 204–07.

4. Gay Hendricks, Ph.D., *Conscious Breathing: Breathwork for Health, Stress Release, and Personal Mastery* (New York: Bantam Books, 1995), 112–14.

5. "A Multidimensional Approach to Pain Relief: Case Report of a Patient with Systemic Lupus Erythematosus," The International Journal of Clinical and Experimental Hypnosis 31 (1983), 72–81.

6. William Mundy, M.D., "Imagery as a Cure for Immune Disorders," *Alternative Health Practitioner* (Fall/Winter 1996), 199–206.

7. Ibid.

8. Steven Lock, M.D., and Douglas Colligan, *The Healer Within: The New Medicine of Mind and Body* (New York: Dutton, 1986), 100–114.

Chapter 12: Caring for Your Spirit

1. Larry Dossey, M.D., *Healing Words: The Power of Prayer and the Practice of Medicine* (New York: Harper, 1993), 110.

2. Ibid., 114.

3. Larry Dossey, M.D., *Prayer Is Good Medicine* (New York: Harper, 1996), 91.

4. Ibid., 49.

5. Janet Austin and Richard S. Maisiak, "Health Outcome Improvements in Patients with Systemic Lupus Erythematosus Using Two Telephone Counseling Interventions," Arthritis Care and Research 9 (1996).

6. Harriet Beinfield and Efrem Korngold, *Between Heaven and Earth: A Guide to Chinese Medicine* (New York: Ballantine Books, 1991), 383.

7. Andrew Weil, M.D., *Spontaneous Healing* (New York: Ballantine Books, 1996), 214.

Index